Protecting Children from Abuse and Neglect in Primary Care

Protecting Children from Abuse and Neglect in Primary Care

Edited by

Michael J. Bannon

Associate Dean in Postgraduate Medicine
London Deanery
20 Guilford Street
London WC1N 1DZ

and

Yvonne H. Carter

Department of General Practice and Primary Care
Basic Medical Sciences Building
Queen Mary and Westfield College
London

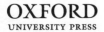

OXFORD
UNIVERSITY PRESS

OXFORD
UNIVERSITY PRESS

Great Clarendon Street, Oxford OX2 6DP

Oxford University Press is a department of the University of Oxford. It
furthers the University's objective of excellence in research, scholarship,
and education by publishing worldwide in

Oxford New York

Auckland Bangkok Buenos Aires Cape Town Chennai
Dar es Salaam Delhi Hong Kong Istanbul Karachi Kolkata
Kuala Lumpur Madrid Melbourne Mexico City Mumbai Nairobi
São Paulo Shanghai Taipei Tokyo Toronto

Oxford is a registered trade mark of Oxford University Press in the UK
and in certain other countries

Published in the United States by Oxford University Press Inc., New York

A catalogue record for this title is available from the British Library

Library of Congress Cataloging in Publication Data
(Data available)

ISBN 0 19 263276 0 (Pbk)

10 9 8 7 6 5 4 3 2 1

Typeset in Minion by
Integra Software Services Pvt. Ltd, Pondicherry, India
www.integra-india.com
Printed in Great Britain
on acid-free paper by Biddles Ltd, Guildford and King's Lynn

Foreword

Primary care is for everyone. People of all ages with all problems see their general practitioners and practice nurses as their first port of call, their first contact with the National Health Service and social care. Some people who we see are particularly vulnerable and cannot argue for their own care without support from health professionals. In particular, those from deprived areas, the elderly and those with mental health issues spring to mind.

However, a large group of vulnerable people are children. Where they have supportive, caring parents or guardian children have a natural advocate and protector – where such support is missing the primary care team becomes a key element in that child's care. Most children are not abused or neglected. However, many experience bullying, bereavement, family break-up, movement from community to community, and personal failures.

All children, therefore, deserve access to a carer outside their family, someone who they can turn to for confidential help and advice, someone who has their best interests at heart. All general practitioners, practice nurses and community nurses must understand this need and must have the skills to fulfil the role. They require training and education. They must recognize early signs of distress, neglect or abuse and know how to respond.

Yet this is an area in which many general practitioners feel ill at ease. Not only is there an information and skill gap, but there are more emotional issues. Putting aside our natural tendency to prefer not to believe that children in our area could be abused, the exploration of suspicions has implications that are not present in normal consultations.

We try to practise medicine in the family setting. Protecting one family member may involve distancing oneself from other family members. One doctor–patient relationship may have to take precedence over others. The involvement of the law and predetermined local procedures adds to the perceived difficulties.

However, this is not an area in which doctors and nurses have a choice. We have an obligation to vulnerable children and that is an obligation we must discharge. We do not do so alone. This is quintessentially an area in which teams come together to ensure a holistic, sympathetic but effective response. Individual clinicians do not have to bear responsibility alone.

This book addresses these issues. It does so with sagacity and imagination. The reader – and all primary care team members would benefit from it – is offered facts, skills, attitudes and insights to help in this difficult area. We can all do child protection better – let us use this book to achieve that aim.

Mike Pringle
June 2002

Preface

Why this book was written

Child abuse and neglect seem to be always in the news, whether in the media or in the medical press. It represents a difficult and complex subject, capable of provoking a variety of feelings from health professionals including distaste, disbelief and perhaps a reluctance to become involved. However, the protection of children from abuse or neglect should represent a shared responsibility of all those who care for children and their families.

Both of the editors have in the past been members of Area Child Protection Committees (as designated paediatrician and GP representative). As a result, we became aware of the issues surrounding the role of primary care and the protection of children from abuse and neglect. In particular, we knew that the apparent reluctance of GPs to become involved in the child protection process was a subject of concern for Social Services. At the same time, we were conscious of the challenges faced by primary care workers in this most difficult area of clinical practice. We could therefore see the argument from both sides. As clinicians with regular contact with children and their families, we were also conscious of the devastating impact of abuse on child development and welfare. Research undertaken by us confirmed that the involvement of the primary health care team, particularly the GP, was complex, misunderstood and fraught with difficulty. Having explored these issues by further research and discussion with key informants, we have formed certain conclusions on the subject. We thought it important to share these findings with a larger audience of primary health care professionals.

There was a need therefore for an information resource that would enable GPs of all levels of experience and other members of the primary health care team to gain a greater insight with respect to their role in child protection. At the same time, we hoped that social workers and leaders of primary care organizations would also find this of benefit in this respect.

We have initially followed more traditional paths with respect to some of the contents. Leading authorities have therefore contributed chapters on the following aspects of child abuse: epidemiology, legal aspects, clinical presentation and effects of categories of abuse, overview of the child protection process and what to do and say when abuse presents itself to practitioners.

However, we have attempted to broaden the focus of the book:

1 In recognition of the multicultural nature of our communities, there is a chapter that specially addresses relevant cultural issues and another compares child protection systems across different countries.

2 As GPs provide care for all family members, we have dealt with the important subjects of domestic violence and its relevance to child abuse, adult survivors of abuse and looked after children.

3 Worldwide, there is a palpable move towards a primary care led health service and the UK is no exception. Dr Bastable has explored the challenges in this context that Primary Care Trusts will face as they attempt to address children's needs.

4 Professor Browne and Dr Hamilton have looked to the future and consider the frequently overlooked issue of how abuse may be prevented.

On reading these chapters together, several themes become apparent. It is of interest that our contributors, writing independently, have identified numerous recurring themes, the more interesting being as follows:

1 We are repeatedly reminded of children's rights and the paramountcy principle that requires us to place the welfare of children above all other consideration. Several authors allude to the UN Convention on the Rights of the Child (1989) in this respect.

2 The need for training of all primary health care professionals at all levels, separately within their own discipline and together as a team is also emphasized by several authors. Furthermore, there is a recognized need for *education* (which positively influences attitudes) as well as *training* (which ensures that professionals recognize abuse and know what to do).

3 There is a palpable mood of optimism with respect to the positive impact that the newly emerging Primary Care Trusts in England (and their equivalent in other countries within the UK) could effect within this area. Child protection would then be seen as part of a broader children's agenda that would include disability and health promotion.

On reviewing the chapters some time after they had been originally commissioned, we are immediately aware of a number of limitations of our book. First, while it is recognized that all GPs are part of a larger team of professionals and support staff, there is a tendency to consider the role and challenges faced by GPs primarily. Perhaps this is not a bad thing, as most primary health care teams are usually led by GPs who are well placed to take a lead on this important subject. Second, rapid change is taking place within both the NHS and health care systems worldwide. One significant development in England has been the development of Workforce Development Confederations (WDCs). These will undoubtedly become significant key players in the child protection process in the future. We will watch the influence of WDCs in this area with interest.

We would like to thank all of the authors for their contributions. There are numerous quotes which give food for thought. Perhaps, the most pervasive is that made by Tom Narducci (Chapter 16):

> If we recognized our shared responsibility . . . we could overcome every block to effectively protecting children that has been identified. We can do it and we should do it. The question is *will* we do it?

Michael Bannon and Yvonne Carter
June 2002

Contents

List of contributors

Michael J. Bannon
Associate Dean in Postgraduate
Medicine
London Deanery
20 Guilford Street
London WC1N 1DZ

Ruth Bastable
General Practitioner
Monkfield Medical Practice
Cambourne
Cambridge CB3 6AJ

Mitch Blair
Reader in Child Health
Imperial College School of Medicine
and Consultant Paediatrician
Northwick Park Hospital
Watford Road
Harrow
Middlesex HA1 3UJ

Kevin D. Browne
Centre for Forensic and Family
Psychology
School of Psychology
University of Birmingham
Edgbaston B15 2TT

Yvonne H. Carter
Department of General Practice &
Primary Care
Basic Medical Sciences Building
Queen Mary & Westfield College
London E1 4NS

Fran Clift
Parmer, Weightman Vizards
High Holborn House
52-54 High Holborn
London WC1V 6RL

Christopher Cloke
Head of Child Protection Awareness
NSPCC National Office
42 Curtain Road, London EC2A 3NH

Leslie L. Davidson
Director, National Perinatal
Epidemiology Unit
Institute of Health Sciences
Old Road Headington
Oxford OX3 7LF

Geoff Debelle
Consultant Community Paediatrician
The Birmingham Children's Hospital
Steelhouse Care
Birmingham B4 6NH

Anna Gupta
Lecturer
School of Social Work
University of Leicester
107 Princes Road East
Leicester LE1 7LA

Alyson Hall
Consultant Child & Adolescent Psychiatrist
Emanuel Miller Centre for Families and
Children
Gill Street, London E14 8HQ

Catherine E. Hamilton
Centre for Forensic and Family Psychology
School of Psychology
University of Birmingham
Edgbaston B15 2TT

Enid Hendry
Head of Child Protection Training
NSPCC National Training Centre
3 Gilmour Close
Beaumont Leys, Leicester LE4 1EZ

Rachael Hetherington
Associate Research Fellow
Department of Health and
Social Care
Brunel University Uxbridge,
Middlesex UB8 3PH

Chris Hobbs
Consultant Paediatrician
St James University Hospital
Beckett Street
Leeds LS9 7TF

Neil R. Jackson
GP Dean
London Deanery
20 Guilford Street
London WC1N 1DZ

Jocelyn Jones
Director
School of Social Work
University of Leicester
107 Princes Road East
Leicester LE1 7LA

Professor Margaret A. Lynch
Professor of Community Paediatrics
Guy's, King's and St Thomas' School
of Medicine
Newcomen Centre
Guy's Hospital
St Thomas' Street
London SE1 9RT

Mary Mather
Consultant Community Paediatrician
Greenwich Primary Care
(NHS) Trust
Woolwich
London SE18 6QR

Alison Mott
Consultant Community Paediatrician
Dept of Community Child Health
Landsdowne Hospital
Sanatorium Road
Canton Cardiff CF1 8UL

Tom Narducci
NSPCC National Training Centre
3 Gilmour Close
Beaumont Leys, Leicester LE4 1EZ

Melanie Pace
NSPCC National Training Centre
3 Gilmour Close
Beaumont Leys
Leicester LE4 1EZ

Ximena Poblete
Consultant Paediatrician
Northwick Park Hospital
Watford Road
Harrow Middlesex HA1 3UJ

Professor Mike Pringle
Professor of General Practice
Division of General Practice
School of Community Health Sciences
University of Nottingham
Nottingham, UK
NG7 2RD

Anne-Marie Slowther
Research Fellow
47 Lonsdale Road
Summertown, Oxford OX2 7ES

Wendy Thorn
Designated Nurse
Child Protection Clinical Effectiveness Team
Caryl Thomas Clinic Headstone Drive
Wealdstone HA1 4UQ

Chapter 1

Overview of child abuse and neglect

Ximena Poblete

Child abuse and neglect: how much have we learnt?

The evidence from research carried out during the last thirty years has placed child abuse and neglect within the most serious health conditions affecting children. Increased knowledge on risk factors has helped to unravel a complex process, whereby child abuse is seen to occur as the result of an interaction between parents, a vulnerable child and a family's social and cultural environment (Belsky 1993). There is enough research evidence to confirm the devastating effects that abuse has on a child's overall health and we recognize the long-term effects of maltreatment, from childhood through to adulthood.

Information from the National Society for the Prevention of Cruelty to Children (NSPCC) (Creighton 2001) reveals that 100 children die each year from abuse and that infants under 12 months of age are four times more likely to be homicide victims than the rest of the population, with at least one being killed every fortnight. According to the Department of Health statistics for England (Department of Health 1999), between 1997 and 1998 there were 30,000 children newly placed on Child Protection Registers and 78,200 children looked after by local authorities in foster homes and children's homes. Children whose names are placed on Child Protection Registers are known to have suffered abuse over a period of time and are likely to show impaired health or development as the result of their ill-treatment. The impact of abuse on children's mental health is confirmed by data gathered on children aged 5 to 12 years, at time of entering local authority care, which shows that at least 50% of children admitted to residential placements suffer from very high levels of depression and almost 40% have very high levels of conduct disorder (Dimigen *et al.* 1999). Sadly the long-term outcome of *looked after children* is very worrying, as 67% of young people leaving care have mental health problems and almost half of the prison population and young people living rough report having been in care (see also Chapter 17).

The gap between research and practice (1970–2000)

In spite of all the knowledge gathered during these last three decades, child abuse and neglect remain an important cause of mortality and morbidity in childhood and many vulnerable children who have suffered abuse remain at risk of further abuse and a poor outcome in life.

It is well recognized that research findings take several years before leading to a change in clinical practice. In the field of child abuse and neglect this process can take even longer, as the change that needs to take place not only involves the medical and nursing profession, but demands a change in the whole of society. Furthermore, a change in our individual clinical practice may require a change that extends beyond our professional role and into our personal lives. Postulating child abuse as a differential diagnosis can be as difficult today as it was for colleagues thirty years ago, as it challenges our beliefs and may require us to consider the 'unthinkable'. Clinical experience and research have shown that the boundaries of abuse are not fixed, so that the unthinkable can always defy our beliefs and values. Increasing awareness of sexual abuse in the 1980s followed the recognition of physical abuse in the 1960s and 1970s. Knowledge that is more recent has exposed the different faces of fabricated or induced illness, brought to light the child sexual abuse inflicted by mothers and described abuse from one child to another child.

The acknowledgment by health professionals that child abuse is not a rare event, that it can occur in all social classes, can potentially involve any parent and that all children can be vulnerable to abuse, requires a shift in professional, cultural and social values. These issues may lead to a significant bias in the diagnosis of child abuse, as they will lead to a systematic deviation from the recognition of the 'true state' of child abuse and neglect. Some of these dilemmas can be immense for primary health care professionals, who have the responsibility to care for the health needs of both parents and children; when the diagnosis of suspected child abuse involves doubting the parent, disregarding the history, revising the notion of confidentiality and finally balancing the rights of the parents against the rights of the child.

In search of a clear diagnostic definition of child abuse

The challenge faced by health professionals in the recognition and management of child abuse is made even more complex by the lack of a clear 'diagnostic' definition. Child abuse, defined as an act of commission or omission, which threatens a child's well-being, is determined by what is considered to be socially acceptable within society at a given time. Child abuse can therefore be perceived to lie within a continuum of child rearing practices, which may vary within a culture and from one culture to another. Reaching a consensus of opinion can sometimes be a difficult task for professionals, in particular when living in a multicultural society like the one we have in the United Kingdom; what may be perceived to be an acceptable rearing practice by people in one culture, may be considered to be abusive by people in another. Nevertheless, despite some differences, there is a 'cultural consensus' on the core nurture required by children to grow up and develop into mature adults. Most governments, representing most cultures in our world, have agreed that children have universal rights through their ratification of the Convention on the Rights of the Child (UNICEF 1989). The Convention, which sets international standards on the rights and protection of children, was adopted by the General Assembly of the United Nations in 1989 and ratified by 191 out of the 193 states, excluding the United States of America and Somalia. The Convention highlights children's right to grow up in an environment where their overall needs are met and their safety ensured. Through the recognition that children can have a clear understanding of their circumstances and can make a positive contribution to their upbringing, the Convention also acknowledges the rights of children to be empowered and to be consulted on matters which affect their lives, with due regard to their age and understanding.

The Children Act 1989: the concept of significant harm

In the United Kingdom the Children Act 1989 (Department of Health 1991) has brought into the legal system the principles underpinning the Convention on the Rights of the Child. It acknowledges that the welfare of the child is paramount, that children must be listened to and that all children should have the right to grow up within their families, in an environment which promotes their health and safety (Table 1.1). The Children Act recognizes that child abuse should be addressed within the wider context of child protection, with a focus on prevention strategies and early interventions, where the safeguard of a child's well-being is not the sole responsibility of parents, but also of governments and the community as a whole. The Act acknowledges that there are many children 'in need', children who are growing up in vulnerable families,

Table 1.1 The recognition of children's rights

The UN Convention on the Rights of the Child 1989	The Children Act 1989
World declaration on the survival, protection and development of children	Legislation in the United Kingdom
The well-being of children is paramount	The welfare of the child is paramount
The family has the primary responsibility for the nurturing and protection of children from infancy to adolescence.	'Parental responsibility' gives parents clear rights and duties and is only lost when a child is adopted.
For the full and harmonious development of their personality, children should grow up in a family environment, in an atmosphere of happiness, love and understanding. Governments should support the efforts of parents.	Wherever possible, children should be brought up and cared for within their own families. Health professionals have a duty to work together with local authorities to support families and children 'in need'.
Every effort should be made to prevent the separation of children from their family.	Children 'at risk' of harm are also children 'in need'. Local authorities have a general duty to safeguard and promote their welfare and safety in partnership with parents.
Children have the right to be listened to and participate in decisions which affect their lives.	Children should be kept informed about what happens to them and should participate when decisions are made about their future. Courts will have regard for the wishes and the feelings of the child.'

where they will not access their life chances without the support of public agencies. Therefore, local authorities are given statutory responsibilities to assess the needs of children growing up facing social or family disadvantage to enable appropriate delivery of services. Health professionals are expected to work in partnership with local authorities, following the guidelines from the Department of Health which identify clear roles and responsibilities for commissioners and providers within the health service (Department of Health 1995).

Sadly, it is estimated that out of the 12 million children in England, 4 million are growing up in vulnerable families and 600,000 children are likely to be known to social services at any one time (Department of Health 1999). These figures represent a huge challenge for local authorities, as almost by definition, children in need are likely to suffer extra-familial neglect without the appropriate support from services. However, the definition of child abuse and neglect is not focused on the risk of extra-familial maltreatment, but on that inflicted by parents or carers. The Children Act defines children 'at risk' from abuse as those vulnerable children who are suffering or are likely to suffer 'significant harm'; harm being defined as ill-treatment or impairment of health or development, which is attributable to poor parental care. The Act, which aims to tackle definite or likely abuse, relies on 'measurable' adverse effects of ill-treatment and does not identify clear thresholds of concern, offering a very broad definition of child abuse, where the quality of parental care is guided by the care that it would be reasonable to expect a parent to give. The concepts of 'reasonable' parenting and 'significant harm' are left to the judgment of professionals, who may have difficulty identifying objective thresholds of abuse and may encounter great frustration searching for evidence of ill-treatment.

The view on what constitutes 'reasonable' parenting will be influenced by the care known to be given by the majority of parents to their children, which unfortunately may not always acknowledge children's needs. In a recent study over 90%, both of mothers and fathers in two-parent families, reported using physical punishment on their children: 24% of mothers and 18% of fathers reported hitting or smacking their children weekly or more often. Parents were more likely to hit or smack younger children, so that 52% of one year old children were punished in this way (Nobes and Smith 1997).

'Reasonable parenting' will also be influenced by our perception of the parents themselves, their vulnerability and their individual circumstances. What may be considered to be, in 'normal' circumstances, completely inappropriate adult behaviour towards a child, may be perceived as reasonable behaviour under stressful circumstances. A vulnerable parent who lives in poor and overcrowded housing conditions may be perceived as using 'reasonable chastisement' when using physical or emotional punishment to control their child's dangerous behaviour, whereas the same actions on a well-behaved child whose parent is not perceived to be under stress may be considered to be 'unreasonable' and abusive. Therefore, the perception of reasonable parenting may be subjectively determined by a parent and/or child's vulnerability rather than by a child's needs. A definition of child abuse built upon the unmet needs and rights of a developing child, regardless of circumstances, would provide a more objective guidance that would help towards an early recognition of abuse.

The recognition of child abuse and neglect

The early recognition of childhood maltreatment should be a priority for all health professionals caring for children. The same diagnostic process should be followed as with a traditional medical illness. Known risk factors should alert us to the possibility of child abuse and the history given by the parent, together with our findings on physical examination, should guide us towards an accurate diagnosis. In many cases the clinical presentation and/or the pattern of the injuries will strongly point to child abuse as a differential diagnosis, although more often a concern of abuse may emerge as a 'weaker' diagnostic hypothesis that needs to be explored further. Unfortunately, the diagnostic medical model does not appear as useful as with other health problems. The parental history cannot always be relied on; furthermore, it may obscure, rather than help us, clarify the nature of symptoms and physical signs. The absence of physical signs on examination cannot lead to reassurance, as the majority of children who suffer abuse will have no visible signs on general examination. Medical investigations, so helpful in the diagnosis of other serious medical problems, will help in a very small proportion of cases, either by ruling out an organic problem which can be confused with abuse or by exposing evidence of physical abuse, usually in the more complex and serious cases. An allegation of abuse made by the child is now recognized as the single most important diagnostic sign and evidence of abuse. Unfortunately, abused children rarely disclose their abuse and many victims of child abuse present and disclose their maltreatment only as adults.

The absence of a reliable history and the difficulty of assessing the impact of ill-treatment on a child challenges early diagnosis, in particular when it involves the more unthinkable forms of abuse. While there has been an increasing awareness of physical abuse, neglect and emotional abuse, the unwillingness and difficulties of considering child sexual abuse and fabricated or induced illness remain. Like other conditions in health, the more complex the clinical presentation, the more difficult it will be to reach the right diagnosis. However, while the knowledge acquired through theoretical learning and clinical experience may be useful when considering other complex diagnosis, this knowledge may not always help us in the diagnosis of complex child abuse. The more complex the form of abuse, the more difficult it may be to believe it can occur, in particular in a 'normal looking family'. The acknowledgement that any child can be vulnerable to abuse is difficult to accept, in particular for primary health care professionals who are responsible for a given community of patients.

The emotional harm of child abuse

Emotional abuse is at the heart of all forms of abuse. Unfortunately, we have not yet developed the skills or the tools which enable us to easily assess the impact of abuse on a child's behaviour or emotional well-being. Therefore the emotional damage suffered by the majority of children as the result of child abuse and neglect may remain unseen throughout their childhood. Although many abused children will find the resilience required to achieve normal development, research findings have

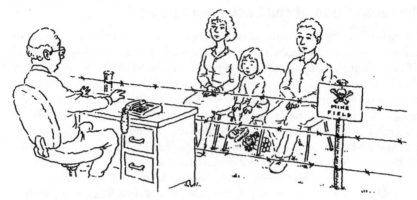

Figure 1.1 The emotional harm of child abuse.

confirmed that many abused children who appear 'well and happy' should be seen as going through a 'latent' stage of an emotional disorder, which may manifest itself later on in their lives (Figure 1.1). The lack of symptoms or signs from abuse on normal children should give no reassurance, as it is well recognized that the impact of a child's ongoing abuse may become visible, for the first time, during adolescence, through a teenagers' defiant behaviour, school truancy or mental health problems. Primary health care professionals may gain insight into a child's experiences of abuse, and develop understanding of the long-term effects of emotional harm through the tragic presentation of young people and adult survivors, who may present with a wide range of physical and mental health problems. The most damaged children and young people may put themselves at serious risk of their own actions, developing self-harming behaviour, becoming the victims of drug and alcohol abuse, youth violence or childhood prostitution.

The role of primary care: addressing conflicting needs

Primary health care professionals are more likely than other health professionals to develop an insight into the social disadvantage and isolation faced by many vulner-able families. In the context of primary health care, balancing the needs and rights of parents against those of their children may become an ongoing challenge, in particular when parents are known to be making efforts to care for their children. Parents who have themselves been abused as children may approach their general practitioners in need of long-term psychological support and immense understanding to help them through the fears and anxieties presented by their own parenthood. Health visitors can gain knowledge of families in their home setting and are ideally placed to identify early signs of stress or potential abuse. Regular discussions of vulnerable families within a primary health care team can help professionals clarify their views, share their concerns and put in place preventative measures to address issues and provide early support to vulnerable families. The wide range of skills and resources within multidisciplinary primary care teams can help to develop management strategies

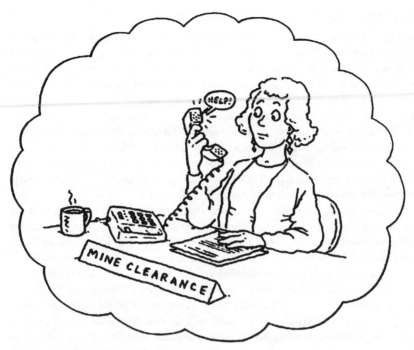

Figure 1.2 Seeking advice in child abuse.

aiming to address the needs of parents and children. All members of primary health care teams should have easy access to named health professionals for discussion and advice on any matters involving child protection (Figure 1.2).

The management of child abuse: working together

In the management of any medical diagnosis, we are guided by the natural history of the disease. We decide on investigations and treatment balancing the positive effects of an intervention against any possible side effects, with the aim of achieving the greatest benefit for our patients. However, in child abuse, only a small proportion of children will require medical treatment; the essential aspect of their management being focused on the investigation of suspected abuse and their need for protection. As stated before, unlike other serious diagnostic hypotheses, child abuse cannot be confirmed or excluded by medical assessments nor investigations alone. The medical information is just one piece of a jigsaw puzzle, which extends beyond the remit of health and can only be completed following a comprehensive assessment, which includes the needs and circumstances of the child and family. Therefore, when a health professional has reasonable cause to suspect that a child is suffering, or is likely to suffer significant harm, a referral to social services becomes an essential aspect of the child's clinical management (Working Together 1999).

Thresholds for referral to social services

A decision to make an early referral to social services will depend on the strength of the diagnostic hypothesis of abuse, on the perceived implications of a mistaken diagnosis and our knowledge on the morbidity and mortality of child abuse. In circumstances when primary health care professionals are aiming to support vulnerable parents, addressing the needs of the child at an early stage may prove difficult. A health visitor, who is trying to support a teenage mother known to have suffered a deprived childhood, may find it difficult to decide when the young mother's limited parenting skills become abusive and fail to meet the needs of her child. On the other hand, a general practitioner treating and caring for a parent with a long-standing mental health problem, may find it hard to decide when the relationship between the parent and the child becomes emotionally abusive for the child.

In the present era of evidence-based interventions we want reassurance that our management decisions, i.e. a referral to social services, will improve outcome and not cause more harm than the presenting complaint. Therefore, health professionals may find it difficult to share information with social services when there is a 'suspicion' of abuse; in particular when confronted with the possibility of a mistaken diagnosis and the negative impact that an intervention may have on a particular family. As with solving other complex health problems, the development of an algorithm can be helpful (Figure 1.3). An algorithm based on objective thresholds of concern that follows agreed procedures within primary care teams, should help professionals to deal more ably with their own individual dilemmas and should also facilitate communication with parents, as it helps to 'depersonalize' the diagnosis and management of abuse.

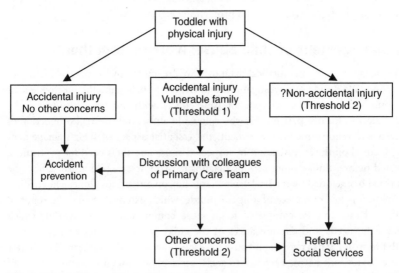

Figure 1.3 Identifying thresholds of concern.

It is important that children who are abused or at risk of abuse access the protection they require from professionals working in close partnership. This is highlighted in Part 8 inter-agency reviews of working together under the Children Act 1989 (cf Chapter 12) looking at the circumstances of children who die from abuse, which sadly bring to light similar lessons each time, emphasizing the need for professionals to share information and work together in the protection of children (Falkov 1996).

Communicating with parents

The concerns of suspected abuse should be shared and discussed with parents, unless this is considered not to be in the child's best interest. Communication with parents in these circumstances is a difficult and often painful task. A vast amount of research has been carried out to help health professionals disclose serious diagnoses to parents in an accessible, comprehensible and supportive way. Unfortunately, much of this does not help when the diagnosis involves suspected child abuse. The personal skills, developed through teaching and clinical experience, which help us to communicate with parents and facilitate the disclosure of other health problems may appear limited when sharing our concerns of possible abuse. Nevertheless, talking to parents is an essential aspect of the management of child abuse, as it is important that parents understand the facts which raise professional concern and that they receive information on the process of referral and involvement of social services. Parents should also be given an opportunity to ask questions and discuss their concerns and anxieties arising from the diagnosis of suspected abuse itself and the child protection process that will follow.

Working towards prevention of child abuse

It is widely acknowledged that child abuse should be seen within the wider context of children 'in need', where parents are supported to meet the needs of their children. Primary care professionals already contribute greatly to the prevention of child abuse and neglect through their time spent dealing with the needs and emotional health issues of parents, alleviating fears and anxieties and making referrals to appropriate support services. Working together between professionals from all agencies caring for children should contribute to the early recognition and management of child abuse, and should help to develop interventions that can ensure the best outcome for children. The ethos of primary health care, based on the promotion of family health through understanding the needs of each member of the family, is an essential contribution to the multi-agency management of children suspected to have suffered or who are likely to suffer abuse. Joint training and the inter-agency commissioning, planning and delivery of services for vulnerable children, should enable us to develop professional relationships based on mutual understanding and trust which will strengthen our services for all children.

Listening to children

The Children Act states that children's wishes and feelings should be acknowledged and their views taken into consideration in decisions which affect their lives. However, vulnerable children who are growing up in deprived and neglectful environments or within abusive families may not be able to develop the self-esteem or confidence required to express themselves. Vulnerable children need to become empowered to express their views and become active participants in decisions affecting their lives. Primary health care professionals play a key role in the protection of children, and are uniquely placed in the community to provide support to children and their families. Children have the right to a safe and nurturing childhood, to reach adolescence with optimism and to grow into adults who are able to enjoy life and contribute to a community they trust and respect. It is our duty as health professionals to make the protection of their rights our business.

References

Belsky J (1993) Etiology of child maltreatment: a developmental/ecological analysis. *Psychological Bulletin* 114: 413–34.

Children Act 1989 (1989) London: HMSO.

Creighton S (2001) *Child Protection Statistics*. London: NSPCC.

Department of Health (1999) *Framework for the Assessment of Children in Need and their Families*. London: HMSO.

Department of Health (1995) *Child Protection – Clarification of Arrangements Between the NHS and Other Agencies: Addendum to Working Together Under the Children Act 1989*. London: HMSO.

Department of Health (2000) *Framework for the Assessment of Children in Need and their Families*. London: The Stationery Office.

Dimigen G, Del Priore C, Butler S, Evans S, Ferguson L and Swan M (1999) Psychiatric disorder among children at time entering local authority care: questionnaire survey. *British Medical Journal* 319: 675.

Falkov A (1996) *A Study of Working Together 'Part 8' Reports: Fatal Child Abuse and Parental Psychiatric Disorder*. Department of Health – ACPC Series. London: Department of Health Publications.

Nobes G and Smith M (1997) Physical punishment of children in two-parent families. *Clinical Child Psychology and Psychiatry* 2(2): 271–81.

United Nations (1989) *The Convention on the Rights of the Child*. United Nations, New York.

Working Together to Safeguard Children (1999) A guide to inter-agency working to safeguard and promote the welfare of children. London: HMSO.

Illustrations by Michael Renouf.

Chapter 2

The child protection process

Melanie Pace

People and agencies will not necessarily collaborate just because someone tells them to work together ... The motivations to work together may be different; the skills, capacities and competence to do so may vary, as does the degree to which they can, in fact, be directed to do so.

(Hallett 1993)

This chapter will guide health professionals through the child protection process in steps from identification, reporting, investigation and intervention. At each stage in the process the law/guidance available will be outlined, and the anxieties/dilemmas for health professionals explored. The chapter will focus on the personal/professional responses to the child protection systems and the perspective of the child/young person. It is aimed at facilitating reflection on how we respond to child protection concerns and why it may be that a mandate to respond of itself cannot be relied upon to ensure multi-agency cooperation.

Detailed information about child abuse, signs and indicators, roles and responsibilities etc. is contained elsewhere in this book. This chapter will, therefore, focus on the process of child protection systems, the potential blocks to implementation and the requirement that, above all else, professionals keep the welfare of the child above all other consideration.

Comparisons will be drawn with regard to the current UK systems and those used in other European Countries (France, Germany and Finland). These comparisons will be limited to some of the legislative differences in the definitions of abuse and the mandate to report. For most health professionals it is the initial elements of the process that will impact on their practice and their responsibilities. Differences in legislation reflect the cultural and social principles of European Union member states, in particular their values and beliefs about the place of the child in society. As I will show, there are varying definitions of violence, differences in the age of consent and in the obligation to report child protection concerns.

Principles of the child protection process

Child protection processes are governed by a legislative framework, supported by professional guidance, based on a set of values and beliefs around childhood, the rights of the child and the rights of the family and community.

These principles are most pertinently identified in the United Nations Convention on the Rights of the Child.

♦ Created over a period of ten years with the input of representatives from different societies, religions and cultures, the Convention was adopted as an international human rights treaty on 20 November 1989.

♦ Built on varied legal systems and cultural traditions, the Convention on the Rights of the Child is a universally agreed set of non-negotiable standards and obligations. It defines the basic human rights of all children. These rights include the right to protection from abuse and exploitation (Article 19).

♦ Those States that are party to the Convention are obliged to develop and undertake all actions and policies in the light of the best interests of the child (Article 3).

♦ The Convention on the Rights of the Child (Article 12) acknowledges the balance between the rights and responsibilities of families on the one hand and the increasing capacity of children, through growth in maturity and understanding, to exercise control over their lives. The recognition of children as participants in the child protection process and not as objects of concern raises issues around consent, disclosure and confidentiality that will be examined later in this chapter.

The current legislative framework for child protection in England (Children Act 1989) is based on the principles of the United Nations Convention. The Act is supported by a set of inter-agency guidelines, 'Working Together to Safeguard Children' (Department of Health 1999). This guidance sets out a framework for assessing children in need (including those in need of protection). This assessment framework draws on all agencies knowledge and understanding to develop an accurate picture of a child's needs based on the child's developmental needs, the parenting capacity to respond to those needs and the wider family and environmental factors. 'Working Together' states that:

> If child protection processes are to result in improved outcomes for children, then effective plans for safeguarding children and promoting their welfare should be based on a wide-ranging assessment of the needs of the child and their family circumstances.
>
> (Department of Health 1999)

Finally, it is important for all authorities involved in child protection systems to be aware of the implementation of the Human Rights Act (1998). This Act came into force in October 2000. The Act aims to make the rights entrenched in the European Convention for the Protection Of Human Rights and Fundamental Freedoms accessible within the English legal system. Article 8 of the Convention reads:

1 Everyone has the right to respect for his private and family life, his home and his correspondence.

2   There shall be no interference by a public authority with the exercise of this right except such as is in accordance with the law and is necessary . . . for the prevention of disorder or crime, for the protection of health or morals, or for the protection of the rights and freedoms of others.

The relevance to health and social care professionals is that they have a duty to consider the impact of their actions. For example, the disclosure of information may breach an individual's human rights to privacy. If so, is this breach overridden by the needs of the other, for example, the child's rights to protection from harm. Professionals must therefore be satisfied that any decision to disclose information to a third party can be seen to be in the best interest of the child and in support of their human rights. This is explored further in this chapter in the section dealing with reporting concerns.

European perspective[1]

France has a complex system of child protection. The legislative framework is governed by Law No. 89–847 of 10 July 1989 Concerning The Prevention Of Ill Treatment Of Minors And The Protection Of Children. There is no official definition of child abuse within this law, although abuse is mentioned, nor is there any law forbidding adults from physically punishing children. Poilpot (1998) advises that those working in France should be guided by the definition given by the National Observatory for decentralised social Action (1993): 'An abused child is one who is the victim of physical violence, mental cruelty, sexual abuse or severe negligence having serious consequences for his physical and psychological development'.

This definition is not far removed from the English use of significant harm and the Working Together Guidance. There is a two-tier child protection system, administrative and judicial, with the role of the judiciary being far reaching.

In Germany, general provisions for child welfare are found in Basic Law, Art. 6 para. (2): 'The care and the upbringing of children is a natural right of parents and a duty primarily incumbent on them. The community is responsible for ensuring that they perform this duty'.

This is also similar to the Working Together Guidance (Department of Health 1999) which refers to parents being supported by 'friends and family and the wider community' (S1.3) and the need for all agencies and professionals to share responsibility to promote children's well-being and safeguard them from significant harm (S1.10). Where Germany and England differ is that the Children Act (1989) moved away from the notion of parent's rights to the concept of parental responsibility. Parental responsibility diminishes as the child acquires sufficient understanding to make his own decisions *Gillick* v. *West Norfolk and Wisbech Area Health Authority* AC112 (1986).

In Germany the definition of child abuse is drawn from a booklet published by the Federal Ministry For Family Affairs in the 1980s: 'Any active or deliberate action or

[1]   See Chapter 19 for further treatment of this subject.

omission which might cause harm or even the death of a child'. Abelmann-Vollmer (1989) notes that the concept of child abuse is recognized as part of a socio-psychological phenomenon, including gender, culture and political issues. There is a lack of clarity with respect to parent's physical punishment of children. Within the Civil Code there is a parent and Child Section 1631 (subsection 2) 1997 which states 'Educational measures offending dignity, especially physical and psychological abuse, are prohibited.' This does not give clear guidance on smacking and is therefore similar to English legislation and guidance. There has been ongoing debate about the issue of parents using physical punishment and the question of what is reasonable chastisement.

Finland offers a marked contrast to France and Germany in its views on the rights of the child with respect to physical chastisement. Sariola and Launis (1998) point out that with the Child Custody and Right of Access Act in 1984, Finland became the second State in the world to prohibit corporal punishment of children. As a result of this legislation, the provisions of the Penal Code on abuse are applicable to all custodians who abuse their children physically, 'even if their stated purpose was to punish the child'. Child protection in Finnish legislation is additionally covered in the Child Welfare Act (1983) amended in 1990 and 1991. As in England, this legislation takes the welfare of the child as the primary consideration and emphasizes preventative and supportive measures and services.

It can be seen that, with a combination of state and family responsibility, there are similar themes in the principles underpinning child protection throughout the above mentioned European Member States. Differences reflect the culture of the countries with regard to the balance between parental rights/responsibilities and the rights of the child.

Identification of child protection concerns

Hallett, in her exploration of multi-agency involvement in child protection, identifies how difficulties can begin even at the stage of recognition of child protection concerns:

> One of the points of difficulty ... centres on differing professional perceptions of what constitutes child abuse; what is sufficiently serious to warrant professional concern and intervention and what should be done in consequence.
>
> Hallett (1993)

Working Together (Department of Health 1999) clearly places the responsibility for recognition of potential harm with all whose work brings them into contact with children and families:

> Teachers, school nurses, health visitors, GPs, Accident and Emergency and all other hospital staff should be able to recognise possible indicators of abuse or neglect in children, or situations where a child requires extra support to prevent significant impairment to his or her health or development.
>
> (Department of Health 1999 page 39)

Health professionals are often the first to be aware that families are experiencing difficulties in looking after their children. Health provision should be universal. Most families will have contact with the primary health care team. All young children are allocated Health Visitor support; family GPs are likely to have first hand knowledge of factors that may impair parenting capacity such as poverty, domestic violence, drug/ substance misuse, disability, mental ill health. Members of the Primary Health Care Team also have a role in monitoring child development and the expertise to recognize difficulties.

The first stage in the child protection process is recognition of concerns with regard to the emotional or physical well-being of the child that may be attributable to the care being given or likely to be given. Recognition of child protection concerns is, however, a complex process in itself. It is important to acknowledge the range of emotions, values, attitudes, beliefs, knowledge and skills that may impact on our ability to 'hear' when presented with a child who may have been abused. It is natural to respond to child abuse with feelings that can range from anger to disgust, pity, horror etc. The response may lead to blocking and denial, especially in circumstances where an individual does not have the opportunity to share their thoughts and feelings. Values and attitudes about abuse can effect an individual's responses to the child and carers. It may be that you feel contempt for the adults yet they may also be your patients, it is possible that you feel some sympathy that seems misplaced, and you may simply not be sure what to feel. Continuing your professional relationship may seem problematic and yet these feelings have to be managed.

A child may ask you to keep a disclosure secret and this can cause a dilemma at what may be perceived as a betrayal of trust. Careful consideration must be given to informing the child of your responsibility to report concerns, in order to reduce the risk of future harm. You may lack skills in communicating with children and may be unaware of the meaning of their words or actions or respond in a way that is silencing rather than facilitative. This may be particularly pertinent in cases where the child has a disability and requires special communication skills. Furthermore, research indicates that disabled children are more vulnerable to abuse and yet this often goes unacknowledged or unseen. Kennedy (1995) points to the nature of society's views on disability as a major factor in why so many might slip through the child protection net.

'Child protection rests on the value and respect which is invested in the child. When the child is judged to be of little value or is not respected, services for that child will be less' Kennedy (1995).

Your own personal sense of identity e.g. race, gender, or ethnicity may have an impact on a child's perceptions of whether they can trust you. If a black child's experience of white authority figures is negative then that child may be reluctant to talk to a white health professional. Children not only recognize difference, they also ascribe value to it. By the time a child has reached the age of three or four years they are developing a growing sense of autonomy and a real need to make sense of the world.

'They are unconsciously absorbing the values of their families and of others in their immediate world. Their **racial** and **cultural** identity is already being determined' McMahon (1992).

No matter how you feel towards individuals of different race, gender, sexuality or disability, the important thing is to be *aware* of the possibility that you may inadvertently silence a child because of how he or she sees you.

Children and young people may have little faith in the adult world. Research carried out into the views of children involved in the child protection process by Butler and Williamson (1994) confirmed that, for many, the responses of adults was unsatisfactory. What emerged from the research was that a substantial number of children and young people had no confidence whatsoever in adult support of any kind. They talked to no one about their lives, concerns or fears. All primary health care professionals need to feel confident both in communicating with children and their carers and in recognizing and responding to possible child protection concerns. The reporting of such concerns requires a sound ethical and professional judgement, and this is the next stage in the child protection process.

Reporting child protection concerns

This is potentially the most contentious part of the child protection process for health professionals. For instance the decision to break patient confidentiality, is a major ethical consideration.

- The General Medical Council has provided guidance entitled *Confidentiality* (1995).[2] This emphasizes the importance of obtaining consent for the disclosure of patient information but makes it clear that there are circumstances in which information may be disclosed without consent. These circumstances include the following.

    If you believe a patient to be a victim of neglect or physical or sexual abuse, and unable to give or withhold consent to disclosure, you should usually give this information to an appropriate responsible person or statutory agency, in order to prevent further harm to the patient.

    (GMC 1995)

- Paragraph 18 of the same document states that it may be necessary to disclose information in the public interest where failure to do so may expose the patient, or others, to risk of death or serious harm. The GMC applies this disclosure of information both in respect of third parties, such as adults who may pose a risk, and about children who may be the subject of abuse. Similar guidance has been produced by the United Kingdom Central Council for Nursing Midwifery and Health Visiting (UKCC) in their Guidelines for Professional Practice (1996).

- The Human Rights Act (Article 3), prohibits torture, inhuman and degrading treatment and punishment. In cases of children who, by reason of their age and vulnerability are not capable of protecting themselves, Article 3 will potentially impose a positive obligation on the authorities to take preventative measures to protect a child at risk.

- Working Together to Safeguard Children (Department of Health 1999) also sets out the specific role of health within the context of multi agency working.

---

[2] The Department of Health has recently issued guidance on consent.

There is therefore a clear mandate for the reporting of child protection concerns. Each Primary Care Team needs to have procedures linked with Local Area Child Protection Committee guidelines. If there is uncertainty as to whether a child needs a child protection referral, then informal discussions or consultation need to take place between the medical practitioner and the local Social Services Department. The recent shift in emphasis from protection to prevention means that such discussions may result in an initial assessment by the Social Services and a decision taken as to whether a child is in need of services (S17 Children Act 1989) or requires protection from harm (S47 Children Act 1989). The decision as to which route to follow is the primary responsibility of the Social Services Department, working in partnership with other agencies.

Working Together (Department of Health 1999), paragraph 7.31, recognizes the legal framework governing the disclosure of information and the importance of working within carefully worked out information-sharing protocols between agencies and professionals. Child protection concerns should be reported to the local Social Services Department or the police. An emergency duty service for Social Service referrals that need to be made outside normal office hours is in place in every district. Referral information needs to include the child's date of birth, full name, address, family details and a clear factual description of concerns, what has been said/seen and by whom. For health professionals, as for all involved in the field of child protection, the overriding principle should be the welfare of the child. It needs to be recognized that it is only following the collation of information that an accurate picture of a child's circumstances can be put together and an informed decision made as to the steps required to safeguard his welfare. Therefore, whilst health professionals need to pay cognisance to the right of the patient to privacy, this should be balanced against the rights of the child to protection of health or morals.

European perspective

In France the disclosure of professional information is justified by Article 226–13, in which there is a general obligation to assist minors under fifteen years who are deemed to be suffering from deprivation or cruelty and vulnerable people of any age who by nature of age, disability or illness, are unable to protect themselves. The French criminal code also carries a custodial sentence and heavy fine for failure to take action, or provide information, which could prevent a felony or an offence that causes bodily harm. There is therefore a strong legal mandate to report child protection concerns to the appropriate department.

This mandate contrasts with the position in Germany, where mandatory reporting has never been established. Ablemann-Vollmer (1998) points out that attempts to bring this issue onto the political arena, usually following spectacular cases of child abuse, have failed because of the reluctance of professionals and their perspective on ethical considerations.

In Finland the Child Welfare Act mandates the reporting of child protection or child welfare concerns to the child welfare authorities. This mandate applies to local and government authorities and officials.

In all countries, therefore, health professionals will continue to be guided primarily by the principle of the welfare of the child. Decisions to break confidentiality need to be taken sensitively and in consultation with guidance provided by legislation and professional bodies.

Intervention

The next stage in the child protection process concerns the action taken following referral. The health professional who contacts Social Services should confirm referrals in writing. The initial telephone contact should clarify the action the Social Services will be taking and any further steps required of the referrer. Social Services have a statutory duty to respond where a child is suspected to be suffering, or likely to suffer significant harm (S47 Children Act 1989). In all circumstances, following referral there will be an initial assessment to draw together relevant information. The purpose of this assessment is outlined in the Working Together to Safeguard Children Guidance (Department of Health 1999):

> Help provide sound evidence on which to base often difficult professional judgements about whether to intervene to safeguard a child and promote his or her welfare and, if so, how best to do so and with what intended outcomes.

It is significant that the current Working Together Document and the assessment framework were compiled as a response to the recognized deficiencies in the system, under which referrals of concerns would be managed under S47 enquiries and as a result fail to identify need. Gibbons *et al.* (1995) researched the child protection systems and identified the overuse of S47 enquiries which are often to the detriment of the child. Six out of seven children who entered the system at referral were filtered out without needing to be placed on the child protection register. Gibbons concluded that an excess of investigations produced neither protective action nor the offer of any other service. Too many families struggling in bringing up their children were defined as child protection cases rather than as families in which there were children in need.

The shift in emphasis from protection to greater use of S17 of the Children Act may encourage referrals from those medical practitioners who have been reluctant to contact the social services because of their concerns about the nature of the process. Where there is a risk to the life of a child or the likelihood of immediate harm, the social services or NSPCC can take emergency action through making an application to the court for an Emergency Protection Order (S44) (Children Act 1989). In some circumstances, this action may be taken by the police (S46). Orders will only be made if the threshold criteria is met and if the order is deemed necessary to protect the child.

In most circumstances, however, a strategy meeting will be held, involving all relevant agencies, to plan the next stage of the enquiry. It is usual for the referring agency to be invited to this meeting to share information.

The impact of enquiries on families, identified by Gibbons *et al.*, has been acknowledged. Working Together notes that authorities should seek to carry out enquiries in such a way as to minimize distress to the child, and to ensure that families are treated sensitively and with respect. It is only if enquiries substantiate the concerns and the child is judged to be at continuing risk of significant harm that the next stage of the child protection process is invoked. This stage consists of the child protection conference. It is the forum for the sharing of information by practitioners whereby the severity of abuse is assessed and the degree of risk evaluated. The conference is a pivotal part of the process, and health practitioners will often have an important role to play. Humphries and Gully (1999) identify the knowledge that health practitioners might be able to contribute. They look at the information potentially held by General Practitioners, hospital based practitioners, health visitors, community psychiatric nurses and paediatricians, all of whom should attend conferences on children known to them.

> Health practitioners attending must focus on the needs of the child during the conference and give views based not only on their own experience, but also on the needs and wishes of the child and the need to protect that child from future harm.

Other agencies that may attend include the police, education, other members of the family and foster carers. Those attending should be there because they have knowledge of the child or family and can make a significant contribution. It can greatly assist the conference if the professionals provide a written report detailing their involvement with the family, their knowledge of the child's health and development and the capacity of the parents to safeguard and promote the child's well-being. The conference should determine if the child is at continuing risk of significant harm and only in these circumstances will the child's name be placed on the child protection register and a child protection plan drawn up. The principle purpose of the register is to make agencies aware of those children who are judged to be at continuing risk of significant harm. Inclusion of the child's name on the register does not give the local authority any legal mandate to intervene, although the conference may decide that action under the Children Act (1989) is necessary to protect the child. A core group will be formed to develop and implement the plan and this may well include members of the primary health care team, particularly health visitors. The plan should draw up clear objectives linked to the reduction of risk and outlining areas of responsibility for the implementation of agreed action. A date is agreed for the next conference (the review) and the circumstances that may necessitate an earlier conference to be convened. Deregistration should be considered at every review at such time as it is considered the child is no longer at continuing risk of significant harm, has moved to another local authority (they will have the responsibility of convening a conference) or the child has reached 18 years of age.

Summary

This chapter has sought to guide health professionals through the child protection process. The overriding principle is that all those working in the health field have a commitment to protect children, and that their participation in inter-agency procedures is essential if the interests of children are to be safeguarded. Countries that are signatories to the UN Convention on the Rights of the Child and subject to the jurisdiction of the European Court of Human Rights have a responsibility for the safeguarding of the welfare of children. The differences in legislative framework and the definitions of childhood lead to contrasting thresholds for action, but this does not take away the primacy of child protection.

Safeguarding children from harm begins with an understanding of the nature of child abuse and a willingness to recognize it as a possibility. The chapter has not underestimated the importance of medical ethics as they relate to patient's rights to confidentiality, but demonstrated the legal framework under which that right to privacy may be broken.

Doctors can and should seek advice from experienced colleagues. At this stage information can be given without disclosure of the name of the child/family. If a critical threshold of professional concern is reached then concerns must be shared with the statutory agencies. Only these agencies have the authority to investigate and intervene.

All intervention will be on the basis of an initial assessment. A child protection enquiry (S47 Children Act 1989) will only be instigated if the information received by the local authority is deemed to meet the criteria of risk.

The case conference provides the forum for further multi-agency sharing of information (including the views of the child and carers) in order that decisions can be made about the most appropriate steps to protect the child from significant harm. Health professional attendance at Case Conferences, to share relevant information, is of great value to this process. Primary health care teams, particularly health visitors, and community nurses will often have an important role in the ongoing work with the children and their families to reduce the risk of harm and to measure the impact of the interventions on the physical well-being of the child.

In conclusion, the child protection process, in principle, is not complex as it consists of three basic stages: recognition, reporting and intervention. The anxieties and dilemmas that may inhibit the process arise from individual and professional values and beliefs. What is clear however is that there is sufficient guidance to support the full involvement of health care professionals in a process, which is often dependent on their expertise, to safeguard children.

References

Ablemann-Vollmer (1998) Germany, in E Andrikopoulou (ed.) (1998) *Are Children Protected Against Violence in Europe?* Bruxelles: European Forum for Child Welfare.

Butler I and Williamson H (1994) *Children Speak*. London: Harlow.

Children Act (1989) *Great Britain, Laws and Statutes*. London: HMSO.

Concerning the Prevention of Ill-treatment of Minors and the Protection of Children 1989 Law no. 89–487 of 10 July 1989.

Department of Health (1999) *Working Together to Safeguard Children*. London: HMSO.

General Medical Council (1998) *Guidance leaflet: Confidentiality and People under 16*. London.

Gibbons J et al. (1995) *Operating the Child Protection System: A Study of Child Protection Practices in English Local Authorities*. London: HMSO.

Hallett C (1993) 'Working together in child protection', in L Waterhouse (ed.) *Child Abuse and Child Abusers: Protection and Prevention*, Jessica Kingsley.

Humphries L and Gully T (1999) *Child Protection for Hospital Based Practitioners*. London: Whurr.

Kennedy M (1995) Rights for Children Who are Disabled, in B Franklin (1995) *Handbook of Children's Rights*. London: Routledge.

McMahon L (1992) *Handbook of Play Therapy*. New York: Routledge.

NSPCC *Turning Points, a Resource Pack for Communicating with Children*. Module 4, pp. 85–8.

National Observatory for Decentralised Social Action (1993), in E Andrikopoulou (ed.) (1998) *Are Children Protected Against Violence in Europe?* (p. 39) Bruxelles: European Forum for Child Welfare.

Poilpot (1998) France, in E Andrikopoulou (ed.) (1998) *Are Children Protected Against Violence in Europe?* Bruxelles: European Forum for Child Welfare.

Sariola H and Launis M (1998) Finland, in E Andrikopoulou (ed.) (1998) *Are Children Protected Against Violence in Europe?* Bruxelles: European Forum for Child Welfare.

The Finnish Child Custody and Right of Access Act (1983) amended in 1984 and Decree 1994.

The Finnish Child Welfare Act (1983) amended 1990 and 1991.

The German Basic Law Article 6, paragraph 2, sentence 1, in E Andrikopoulou (ed.) (1998) *Are Children Protected Against Violence in Europe?* (p. 39) Bruxelles: European Forum for Child Welfare.

The German Civil Code: Parent and Child Section 1631, subsection 2, revised November 1997.

United Nations (1989) *The Convention on the Rights of the Child*. United Nations: New York.

Chapter 3

Child abuse and primary care

Yvonne H. Carter and Michael J. Bannon

GPs are well placed to identify at an early stage family stress which may point to a risk of child abuse, or to notice in the child indications of significant harm, or likelihood of significant harm.

(Working Together 1999)

General practice and primary care are at the centre of the British National Health Service (De Maeseneer *et al.* 2000). They offer an effective, efficient service that is highly valued by patients. Recently *The NHS Plan* for England has stimulated debate on the core values of general practice, its quality and training, and hence on its ability to deliver high quality patient care (Secretary of State for Health 2000). This chapter will describe the roles of the general practitioner and other members of the primary health care team (PHCT) generally in patient care and more specifically in the detection and management of child abuse.

A definition of the overall role and responsibilities of the general practitioner was agreed in 1969 by the Royal College of General Practitioners (Royal College of General Practitioners 1969). It states:

The general practitioner is a doctor who provides personal, primary and continuing medical care to individuals and families. He may attend his patients in their homes, in his consulting-room or sometimes in hospital. He accepts the responsibility for making an initial decision on every problem his patient may present to him, consulting with specialists when he thinks it appropriate to do so. He will usually work in a group with other general practitioners, from premises that are built or modified for the purpose, with the help of paramedical colleagues, adequate secretarial staff and all the equipment which is necessary. Even if he is in single-handed practice, he will work in a team and delegate when necessary. His diagnoses will be composed in physical, psychological and social terms. He will intervene educationally, preventively and therapeutically to promote his patient's health.

There are over 36,000 general practitioner principals in the UK, with an average list size of just over 1800 registered patients. Although the average list size for each principal is falling slightly in historical trends, the number of consultations per unrestricted principal is rising. Since 1984, the number has risen by nearly 800 per year, to 8,978 consultations in 1996. This means that principals in general practice do 324 million consultations a year. When those with non-principals are included, the number rises to about 350 million consultations with general practitioners per year.

On average, females visit their general practitioner six times a year, and males four times, with an average number of consultations being almost exactly five per year. Both children and the elderly consult more frequently than other age groups. Those under 5 years old consult on average seven times a year as, also, do those aged over 65, compared to three times for those aged between 16 and 44.

In England and Wales 78% of people consulted their general practitioner at least once during the year 1991/92. The General Household Survey in 1998 found that 14% of people had visited their GP in the previous 14 days. When patients visit the surgery to see a doctor, 87% see their own general practitioner or another partner, as opposed to a locum, an assistant or a GP Registrar. The patient's general practitioner or a partner at the practice carries out 82% of home visits.

Patient satisfaction rates with GP consultations are often very high. The NHS Executive's National Survey of NHS Patients (NHS Executive 1999) reported:

> Most (people who had consulted their GP in the previous 12 months) had favourable views of their GP services. In general, most patients felt that their GPs took their opinions seriously, were easy to understand, and kept them well informed about their condition or treatment. 79% considered that their GP knew which treatment was best and 84% that their GP made the right diagnosis most or all of the time. Despite the complexity, import- ance and emotional context of general practitioner consultations, they generate less than 5,000 formal complaints – one for every 70,000 consultations.

Children

The care of children forms a significant part of the general practitioner's and primary health care team's workload. Patients aged fifteen and under comprise 20% of the average general practitioner's list. Care of children under four in particular consti- tutes a considerable part of the workload of a general practitioner. They consult their GP more often and have more home visits than any other age group except for the elderly. The vast majority of children aged fifteen and under receive all their medical care from a general practitioner. The rate of referral to hospital (both in and out patients) for those aged under 15 is 93 per 1,000 consultations, or around 9%. The 1998 General Household Survey found that in the two weeks before interview, 18% of the under 5s and 9% of 5 to 15 year olds had consulted an NHS GP in the 14 days before interview. Figure 3.1 shows where these consultations took place.

Table 3.1 shows that the vast majority of GPs run effective childhood immuniza- tion programmes. In most cases of failure to immunize more than 70% of children, there are societal explanations.

In England and Wales 94% of unrestricted principals are on the child health surveillance list. The figures for Scotland and Northern Ireland are 78% and 92% respectively.

Flexibility in roles should be restricted to individual practices, teams, and primary care groups or trusts. It must include the ability to provide the correct care for each population's characteristics of geography, demography, ethnicity, culture and socio- economics. The same solutions cannot be applied universally, but variations need to be justified on the basis of the needs of that population, and care must be taken to

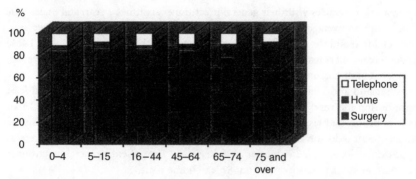

Figure 3.1 Consultations with a GP in the 14 days before interview, by age and site of consultation.

Table 3.1 Target achievements, October 1998, England (Department of Health Statistical Bulletin 1998)

Target	Number	%
Childhood primary immunization		
Those achieving 90%	22,991	84
Those achieving 70%	2,711	10
Total	25,762	95
Pre-school immunization booster		
Those achieving 90%	22,099	81
Those achieving 70%	3,815	14
Total	25,914	95

ensure that every citizen has access to the full range of healthcare professional expertise.

However, these developments must be seen in context. The general practitioner offers the NHS an important range of key attributes and skills. It is not by chance that general practitioners have become central to the health service and are highly respected and supported by their patients (Royal College of General Practitioners 1972).

Over the last twenty years considerable attention has been paid to defining the professional skills and knowledge required for the demonstration of clinical competence. Norman (1985) lists seven categories as a working classification of competency: knowledge, communication skills, history taking, physical examination/technical skills, clinical reasoning/problem solving, decision making and personal values. These skills and attributes are developed during a process of lifelong learning.

Complex clinical skills

A general practitioner is presented with the full range of symptoms, signs and histories in the physical, psychological and social domains. Dealing with these needs high level knowledge, the ability to tolerate uncertainty, the skill to create a safe, effective but not unnecessarily complex management plan, and high-level communication skills. While a protocol may offer guidance in the management of uncomplicated cases, most patients are not uncomplicated and many have extensive comorbidity: angina, hypertension and depression in older patients, for example. The capacity to deploy these skills in a short, ten minute, consultation requires a breadth of biomedical and psychosocial knowledge to be matched to the enormous variety of patient presentations. The complexity of this role, the gatekeeper between perceived illness and disease, must not be underestimated.

Flexibility

Flexibility is a hallmark of the personal care delivered by a general practitioner. GPs reformulate their care to meet the needs of individual patients as they evolve, developing roles to suit the needs of patients. This flexibility is the fundamental key to the high quality and high reputation of most general practices. It offers personally tailored care including the right access to the right parts of the health service when appropriate. Formulaic, protocol-driven care can undermine patient autonomy within the consultation.

Demand management

This results from general practitioners empowering patients to take responsibility for their own care when appropriate, from identifying the right routes through the primary and secondary care services and from taking increasing responsibility for complex patient care in general practice.

Continuity of care

Highly prized by patients. Seeing a doctor who knows the patient and remembers key events in the life of that patient and the family, who will be there subsequently when required and who takes a longer term view of care and its outcomes is an important feature of primary care. Of course, GPs take holidays, retire and move on; not all patients see 'their' GP. But continuity is supported by four crucial features:

1   The lifetime clinical record is retained in general practice. The general practitioner is its guardian although the concept of a patient held and patient involved record is being developed. This record is the key to efficient and safe health care delivery.

2   A population perspective is a key aspect of modern general practice, with health needs assessment, health inequalities and commissioning being addressed.

3   Advocacy on behalf of individual patients, groups of patients and whole communities requires a variety of skills, an overview of the health and social system, the ability to detect and address inequalities and an involvement in commissioning. Good advocacy is based on a shared understanding, which in turn is greatly facilitated by continuity.

4   Team working is now a key feature of general practice, with professional isolation being less common. However the general practitioner fulfils a key role within the team.

These core skills and attributes are fundamental to a good primary care system. From Barbara Starfield's seminal work on international comparisons (1994–1999) and work by Fry and Horder (1995), it is clear that the more primary care orientation there is in a health care system the:

+ higher the patient satisfaction with the health care system
+ lower the overall expenditure on health care
+ better the population health indicators
+ fewer prescribed drugs are taken per head of population.

Why should this be? In British primary care, which is admired throughout the world and visited regularly for insight, we have some valued features that may account for this. These include the registered list; the prevention and management of disease and the gatekeeper role.

Child protection issues in primary care

'Child abuse is the difference between a hand on the bottom and a fist in the face' (Kempe *et al.* 1962). Child protection is a major socio-political issue in the UK. General practitioners, nurses and other staff working in primary care have a key role to play in identifying children who may have been abused, and in initiating protective action.

Recognition of child abuse is not always straightforward, and cases are often missed. Members of the primary health care team need to understand and be able to recognize indicators of child abuse, know what procedures to follow, and feel part of a wider team of professionals involved in child protection.

Clinical practice in the recognition and management of child abuse has evolved over the past 40 years. There has been a widening of the term 'child abuse' from the 'battered baby syndrome' of the 1960s, through emotional abuse and neglect, to sexual abuse and Münchausen syndrome by proxy (see later chapters). *Child abuse* is the label attached to a varied set of actions considered abusive to children. One difficulty for general practitioners and their teams results from differing professional and cultural perceptions of what constitutes child abuse: what is sufficiently serious to warrant professional concern and intervention, and what should be done in consequence?

The diagnosis of child abuse or neglect is a difficult intellectual and emotional exercise for any health professional. It is a distressing subject area of clinical practice, needing time, experience and emotional strength. Full participation demands health professionals to undertake a number of sequential, developmental steps (Figure 3.2). Perhaps the greatest barrier to diagnosis results from an emotional block in the minds of health professionals. A fundamental requirement in this context is the acknowledgement that child maltreatment exists and that it is unfortunately a common phenomenon that has detrimental effects on child welfare and development. Furthermore, primary care staff must accept that child protection work is a responsibility for all health professionals who have contact with children and their families. It follows that there is an obligation on the part of primary care health professionals to develop an adequate awareness of the agreed clinical indicators of child abuse and familiarize themselves with local referral arrangements. Vigilance for the possibility of abuse must be continuously maintained in order that it is promptly recognized. The last step (reporting and subsequent participation in inter-agency intervention) is perhaps the most difficult and raises particular challenges for the primary care doctor.

It must be remembered that the majority of parents who attend a GP's surgery with their children are transparent and open: they are concerned that their children may be ill, or they are attending for routine child health surveillance and promotion. Child maltreatment may present in a variety of ways to the general practitioner:

1 Injuries suggestive of physical maltreatment may be found during a medical examination or routine child health surveillance procedure;

2 Allegations or disclosures of abuse may be made by a child, relative, other carer or neighbour;

3 On occasion, an injured child may be brought to the surgery for treatment;

4 The practice may receive notification of one or more attendances at a local accident and emergency department;

5 Different members of the primary health care team may express concerns about a child's welfare over a period of time.

The history and/or physical findings may be clearly indicative of abuse and demand urgent referral to the statutory agencies. More frequently, the presentation is not so clear-cut and must be considered as one part of an overall picture to be pieced together rather like pieces of a jigsaw puzzle. Table 3.2 (which is by no means exhaustive) summarizes the more common clinical indicators of child abuse by category and also emphasizes the difficulties inherent in making a diagnosis. This list illustrates the difficulties inherent in the identification of child abuse or neglect. Some signs or

Table 3.2 Clinical indicators of abuse by category

Physical abuse	Neglect
Multiple superficial injuries of varying type, size and age	Untreated medical conditions
Delay in seeking treatment	Inadequate compliance with child health surveillance and immunization programmes
Bruises or welts resembling shape of article used to inflict injury	Poor hygiene
Injuries incompatible with given history or child's developmental age	Failure to thrive
Central nervous system injuries in infants	Developmental delay

Emotional abuse	Sexual abuse
Behavioural disturbances	Sexualized behaviours
Poor school performance	Behavioural disturbances
Anxiety	Abrasions/bruises of external genitalia or thighs
Failure to thrive	Sexually transmitted infections
Enuresis/encopresis	

symptoms must be considered more or less as pathognomic of abuse (such as presence of a sexually transmitted infection in a pre-school child) while others (e.g. enuresis) are not so indicative and are found in a wide variety of other and more benign clinical circumstances.

Challenges for primary care

So what are the dilemmas for general practitioners? The following case histories illustrate the difficulties and challenges:

Case one:

A 14-year-old boy attends surgery alone with an upper respiratory tract infection. During the consultation, he tells you that he is also having problems sleeping. He later tearfully discloses that he was sexually abused four years ago by a distant relative but does not want you to tell anyone, including his parents.

Questions:
Can a child of 14 years have autonomy under these circumstances? In this ethical dilemma, do you as a doctor override his perceived autonomy, or do you make a proxy decision on his behalf, believing that as a child he has not yet developed his own autonomy and cannot know what is best for him?

Case two:

During the six-week check, the practice health visitor reports that she has noted some marks around a baby girl's mouth. Mother is aged 18 years, is single and unsupported. She claims that the baby is difficult to feed; that she cries a lot and that she has to hold the baby's mouth firmly in order to ensure that she finishes each bottle feed. Examination reveals a normal, thriving infant who is well cared for.

Questions:
Do you do anything? Feel reassured that the baby seems well apart from the marks which admittedly resemble bruises but are otherwise trivial? Advise the mother that holding a young baby in this way is inappropriate and allow her to go home? Ask the health visitor to arrange further support for the mother? Refer to Social Services?

The decisions facing the GP in these two cases are as follows:

Referral versus doing nothing

The argument for referral would revolve around:

 ◆ Disclosure of previous history sexual abuse by a young adult in case one always requires further action. Doing nothing could result in a perpetrator continuing to abuse other children in the community. Furthermore, previously abused adults would be in need of psychotherapeutic support.

◆ Case two, which highlights a six-week-old baby with trivial injuries but who is otherwise thriving, represents a situation where further investigation is warranted with a view to assessment of risk and provision of family support.
Theoretical reasons for not referring are:

◆ What happens if, following full inter-agency investigation, no convincing evidence of abuse or neglect is found in either case? Families would undoubtedly consider child protection investigative procedures to be intrusive and unpleasant. Surely, in any case the unique relationship with either family would be irretrievably damaged?

◆ Respect of patients' rights with respect to confidentiality is a fundamental guiding principle for primary care (Bannon and Carter 1991).

◆ To whom should referrals be made: Social Services? Police? Paediatrician?

What to do and say

Local guidelines will vary according to precise detail regarding referral and support mechanisms. However, the following universal principles should apply:

1 *Doing nothing* is not an option whenever child abuse is suspected. The outcome for abused children, their families (and also involved health professionals) can be disastrous and is regularly alluded to in the media.[1]

2 *Be aware of local referral procedures.* Most Area Child Protection Committees (ACPCs) have produced simple, A4-sized guidelines for the benefit of all health professionals (including primary care) that include names and telephone numbers of useful contacts as well as specific guidance regarding what to do and say.

3 *Remember the GP's role in child protection.* GPs are *not* expected to be child abuse experts. They are not required to make the definitive diagnosis of abuse or neglect that is more usually undertaken by experienced paediatricians who work closely with other professionals. The GP's role is one of vigilance and reporting.

4 *Think of the paramountcy principle* that dictates that all of your actions must be taken in the best interests of children.

5 *Clarify in your own mind why it is you have suspicions* of abuse or neglect. Is it because of the mother's attitude towards the child or is it because of inconsistencies in the presenting history?

6 *Document who said what, when and where.* Accurate, contemporaneous notes are essential if you have to give evidence as a witness in later court proceedings. If you find injuries that are not in keeping with the history given, then these must also be documented. The child's demeanour and general state of care must also be recorded.

7 *Quickly assess the level of risk of future harm to the child.* Dangerous situations require immediate action. This can be a difficult exercise in practice; hence

---

[1] Climbié doctor admits errors put girl at risk. *Guardian* 12 October 2001.

discussion with Social Services, a consultant paediatrician or more experienced colleague can be very helpful. *Remember: if in doubt, ask.*

8 *Discuss the case with either Social Services or a consultant paediatrician.* Make it clear that you have concerns about child protection. Document the conversation and its outcome in the clinical notes.

9 *Refer to Social Services if there is significant concern of immediate harm to the child.* Make it absolutely clear that you are making a referral because of child protection concerns. Document this in the notes and follow the telephone conversation with a written referral letter.

10 Make arrangements to see the child again, if appropriate.

The above approach may seem prescriptive but it is based upon experience and if followed, could ensure that GPs 'do the right thing', stay out of trouble and, at the same time, help to ensure the safety of children.

With respect to the two case scenarios, the following represent reasonable courses of action:

Case one: 14-year-old boy who alleges previous sexual abuse

1 Document exactly what the boy has said to you and clarify any points as appropriate.

2 It would appear that he is not in immediate risk of significant harm and hence immediate intervention is not needed.

3 The situation is complex and merits further discussion and reflection with respect to the most appropriate way forward. These should be explored with:
   (a) Social Services (who may have relevant information about the extended family);
   (b) Other members of the PHCT who could well have more information to add;
   (c) Child and Adolescent Mental Health Services who can offer support and counselling for the boy.

4 This case represents an example of where confidentiality must be breached in order to ensure the safety and welfare of an individual child and the community in general. All professional organizations and Royal Colleges are united in this view. Hence the patient must appreciate that on this occasion you must share the information he has divulged to you with other parties and that you are doing this in his best interests. GPs should be reassured that they are extremely unlikely to be sued by families for breach of confidentiality when they are acting in the best interest of children (Dyer 1995).

5 It would be useful to make arrangements to see the boy again in the near future in order to ensure that appropriate action has been undertaken.

Case two: Six-week-old baby with facial bruising

1 Document:
   (a) What was found at the six-week check
   (b) What the mother said
   (c) Why the health visitor is concerned

2   This represents a situation where the risk of harm to the infant is high. (Non-ambulant children who are healthy should not have facial bruising).

3   An urgent referral to either Social Services or a consultant paediatrician is mandatory, explaining the reason for your concerns and providing as much helpful background information as possible. (A routine letter for an outpatient opinion is not acceptable here!).

4   You must also explain to the mother why you are making a referral under child protection procedures.

5   It would be useful to arrange to see the baby again in a week's time to maintain contact with the mother.

Child protection requires a good working relationship between the health services, the police and social services. These relationships can be difficult to maintain, and work best if the various professionals meet and work together regularly. In reality, however, this may be impractical, particularly when input from an individual practice may be sporadic over the years. Most health districts now have designated (named) doctors and nurses who are responsible for child protection work. However, the general practitioner may have a difficult task managing the ongoing care of such a family, and may need training and support.

While it is essential to stop and think, and to discuss with colleagues any difficult points in management, it is also necessary to protect children. Families are not always reasonable, do not always take responsibility, and may be very difficult 'partners'. Work in this field requires skill, and is time-consuming and emotionally taxing. The consequences for the child and family if abuse is not recognized or wrongly managed are considerable.

Continuing professional and team development

GPs have a further role to play in the protection of children at primary care level (Dept. of Health 1995). The PHCT is a diverse collection of professionals and administrative staff, all of whom will have some degree of contact with families where there are children. Because of the high prevalence of abuse within our society, they will inevitably encounter children at risk who are in need of protection. All members of the PHCT therefore need child protection training at a level in keeping with their role and level of responsibility (Bannon et al. 1999 a and b). As team leaders, GPs must ensure that all members of the PHCT have an adequate awareness of child protection issues. Sidebotham and Pearce recommended improvements in child protection procedures in accident and emergency departments by means of clear protocols, regular staff training, and increased levels of communication (Sidebotham and Pearse 1997). Similar initiatives could be developed for each PHCT. Implementation of practice-based clinical guidelines across a Primary Care Trust that reflect the policies of local ACPCs would be a step forward. Child protection management within primary care is also amenable to simple audits (see Table 3.3). The specific training needs of general practitioners will need to be addressed by area child protection committees and those involved in postgraduate education (see Chapter 5). However, general practitioners

Table 3.3 Suggested audit topics

Initial checklist
Are all members of the primary health care team aware of local guidelines and revisions?
What are agreed routes of referral for general practitioners?
Does the practice have a copy of the local guidelines and is it up to date?
Who is the designated paediatrician?
Have all doctors and nurses attended a training event within the last two years?
How many practice children are on the child protection register and who are they?
How many case conferences were convened during the past two years concerning children registered with the practice; how many were attended and what were the reasons for non-attendance?

must acknowledge the unique role they could undertake in this area and show further commitment to the protection of children from abuse and neglect (Hallett and Birchall 1992).

> The stakes are high. It is not just the health and well-being of children as they grow up into adults but more than this, the future of the society which the children will construct out of their childhood experiences.
>
> (Hobbs, Hanks and Wynne 1999)

References

Bannon MJ, Carter YH, Barwell F and Hicks C (1999) Perceptions held by general practitioners in England regarding their training needs in child abuse and neglect. *Child Abuse Review* 8: 276–83.

Bannon MJ, Carter YH and Ross L (1999) Perceived barriers to full participation by general practitioners in the child protection process: preliminary conclusions from focus group discussions in West Midlands, UK. *Journal of Interprofessional Care* 13: 239–48.

Bannon MJ and Carter YH (1991) Confidentiality issues in child protection and the general practitioner. *Practitioner* 235: 826–31.

Joint working party of the Department of Health, British Medical Association and Conference of Medical Colleges (1993) *Child Protection: Medical Responsibilities – Draft Guidance*. London.

Cleveland Report (1987) Report of the inquiry into child abuse in Cleveland. London: HMSO.

Lancet, The (1950) Collings Report (Editorial). *Lancet* 1: 547–9.

De Maeseneer J, Hjortdahl P and Starfield B (2000) Fix what's wrong, not what's right, with general practice in Britain. *BMJ* 320: 1616–17.

Department of Health Statistical Bulletin. Statistics for General Medical Practitioners in England: 1988–1998, London: HMSO, 1998.

Department of Health, Child Protection (1995) *Clarification of Arrangements Between the NHS and Other Agencies*. London: HMSO.

Dyer C (1995) Court rules against suing. *BMJ* 311: 75.

Fry J and Horder J (1995) *Primary Health Care in an International Context*. London: Nuffield Provincial Hospitals Trust.

Hallett C and Birchall E (1992) *Co-ordination and Child Protection*. London: HMSO.

Hobbs CJ, Hanks H, Wynne J and Hanks H (1999) *Child Abuse and Neglect: A Clinician's Handbook*, 2nd edn. Churchill Livingstone.

Kempe CG, Silverman FN, Steele BF *et al*. (1962) The battered child syndrome. *Journal of the American Medical Association* **181**: 17–24.

NHS Executive (1999) *National Survey of NHS Patients*. Leeds: NHSE.

Norman GR (1985) Defining competence: a methodological review, in VR Neufield, GR Norman (eds) *Assessing Clinical Competence*. New York: Springer.

Royal College of General Practitioners (1969) The educational needs of the future general practitioner. *Journal of the Royal College of General Practitioners* **18**: 358–60.

Royal College of General Practitioners (1972) *The Future General Practitioner: Learning and Teaching*. London: British Medical Journal for the RCGP.

Royal College of General Practitioners (1996) *The Nature of General Practice*. London: Royal College of General Practitioners.

Sidebotham PD and Pearce AV (1997) Audit of child protection procedures in accident and emergency department to identify children at risk of abuse. *BMJ* **315**: 855–7.

Starfield B and Oliver T (1999) Primary care in the United States and its precarious future. *Health and Social Care in the Community* **7**(5): 315–23.

Starfield B (1994) Is primary care essential? *Lancet* **344**: 1129–33.

Starfield B (1997) The future of primary care in a managed care era. *International Journal of Health Services* **27**: 687–96.

Starfield B (1998) *Primary Care: Balancing Health Needs, Services and Technology*. New York: Oxford University Press.

Secretary of State for Health (2000) *The NHS Plan. A Plan for Investment: A Plan for Reform*. London: The Stationery Office.

Working Together under the Children Act 1989 (1991) London: HMSO.

Working Together to Safeguard Children (1999) London: HMSO.

Chapter 4

Child protection in a multicultural society

Geoff Debelle

Introduction

Many of us have the opportunity and privilege of living and working in a multicultural society. Child abuse occurs in such a society within situations that demand vigilance, understanding and sensitivity. In this chapter, I will draw on an expanding body of literature and experience to provide guidance for primary care practitioners on how to recognize such abuse, how to distinguish it from apparent cultural norms, and how best to contribute to a positive outcome.

Explanations for child abuse and neglect can be considered using an ecological framework. Within such a framework, the social and cultural milieu of the child and family are important factors. I will outline this ecological framework, define what I mean by the terms culture, race and ethnicity and then attempt to define child abuse within a multicultural context. To do this, I will draw heavily on the British and US experience. The key question I will be attempting to answer is this: Is recognition and referral of possible child abuse affected by the cultural context in which it occurs? To put it more starkly: Do thresholds of concern for abuse shift up or down if the child is from a black or minority ethnic group? I will also provide examples where certain culturally sanctioned practices can be mistaken for child abuse.

There is a growing literature on child abuse from many countries and cultural groups (Finkelhor and Korbin 1988) that describes practices such as child labour, incarceration of children, child soldiers and conscripts, child victims of war, and collective victimization such as sexual exploitation. A discussion of these is beyond the scope of this chapter. But it is important to remember that multicultural Britain does have a population of children that have survived such horrors.

The ecological framework

Explanations for child abuse were first sought in the psychopathology of the abuser, then in the faulty interaction between parent and child. Later, socio-economic conditions such as unemployment and poverty were perceived as important factors.

The ecological model (Belsky 1980; Garbarino 1977; Wilson-Oyelaran 1989) attempts to integrate the findings of these earlier perspectives and argues that

> Child abuse can only be understood if it is analysed from a perspective that incorporates the previously disparate levels of analysis, namely the individual, the family, the social environment, and the cultural milieu, and also examines the dynamic interactions both between and within each level.

The ecological perspective emphasizes the place of stress-generating social factors that may predispose to abuse and neglect and the role of formal and informal support mechanisms in moderating such stress at a community or neighbourhood level (Howze and Kotch 1984; Strauss 1980). It also provides a mechanism for understanding the stress generated by cultural change and continuity, which give rise to many potential sources of risk for children, especially in a multicultural context such as the UK, where institutions within the host culture have had a long history oppression of other groups.

Culture, race, and ethnicity

The terms 'race', 'culture' and 'ethnicity' are used in any discourse on multiculturalism and are sometimes used interchangeably. I will clarify how these terms will be used in this chapter.

Race

The term 'race', an arbitrary classification of humans based on a handful of phenotypical features, notably skin colour, has largely been discredited by genetics research (Pfeffer 1998). What people believe about 'race', however, has had profound social and political consequences. A system that sought to allocate people into groups on the basis of a shared biology came to signify the moral, physical and intellectual superiority of the power-dominant white group over subject groups (Brah 1994), and became an instrument of oppression and subordination. Racism and colonialism became part of the shared experience of all black people – the term 'black' is used as an inclusive political term – irrespective of background or country of origin (Robinson 1998). Racism remains a dynamic and potentially destructive force within a multicultural society.

Culture and ethnicity

Culture is characterized by the behaviour and attitudes of a social group. It can be defined minimally as a set of beliefs and ideas that a group draws on to identify and manage the problems of their everyday lives (Hillier and Kelleher 1996).

Ethnicity has been used as both a synonym and as an euphemism for race. It implies one or more of the following: shared origins or social background; shared culture and traditions that are distinctive, maintained between generations, and lead to a sense of group identity; and a common language or religion (Senior and Bhopal 1994). Ethnicity may not correspond to a particular culture. Like race, ethnic differences can be constructed by the dominant group ('us') naming the 'other' by a process that is implicitly ethnocentric (Kelleher 1996). 'Ethnic' becomes shorthand for minority groups whereas white ethnicity, set up as the standard against which all others are measured, is invisible (Pfeffer 1998). The counter argument is that, unlike racial differences, ethnic differences are constructed differences in which groups have a role in naming themselves. This gives the group a sense of community and a focus for political negotiation and struggle against the experience of racism and discrimination (Kelleher 1996). It provides the impetus for multiculturalism, the recognition that peoples of different cultures can flourish in one society and retain their cultural identity (Parekh 2000; Smaje 1995).

Change, adaptability and the multicultural society

Culture and ethnicity are not fixed or immutable but are constantly emerging, especially where there are people from different cultures living side by side, as in multicultural Britain. They will not stay still so that we can count, categorize and describe, for example, the 'Asian' or the 'Irish' family. Yet cultural awareness training manuals and information resources for health professionals are often 'fact files', presenting cultures as fixed products. While they do attempt to help workers to be more aware of, and sensitive to, cultural differences, they may encourage overgeneralization and stereotyping (Pffefer 1998). They should therefore be regarded as guidelines and not absolutes.

Stereotyping

Health professionals must be aware of the ever-present danger of stereotyping when working with people from different ethnic groups. Stereotypes, particularly those relating to child rearing and physical punishment, abound and may alter thresholds for concern to an extent that a child could be placed at risk. Stereotypes may also be expressed from within the group, perhaps giving them currency and legitimacy. How often has one heard: 'physical chastisement is part of our culture'. It may well be. But that is to miss the point, particularly if the effects of the chastisement on the child are severe. (I will return to this theme later).

There are also assumptions made about the existence of extensive family and social networks within 'Asian' communities in Britain. They undoubtedly exist yet a person may be isolated from, or even scapegoated by, other family members (Farmer and Owen 1995). Professionals are required to adopt a position of *investigative curiosity* about an act such as physical abuse. In order to avoid the use of stereotypes, there must also be room for respectful, *exploratory curiosity*, to explore the processes and narratives that shape a person's ethnic identity and give meaning to an act (Burnham and Harris 1996). At any one point, an individual may have many levels of identity and may not wish to be constrained by the presumption of a single ethnic identity. This may be particularly so for second and third generation people whose parents came to Britain as immigrants (Kelleher 1996).

Ethnic self-identity

Ethnic identity depends on an individual's self-identification as well as a group's ethnic designation. These are developmental processes, pertinent for *both* white and black individuals, models for which have been reviewed by Lena Robinson (1998). She links the quality or otherwise of inter-ethnic communication with the stage of self-identity of the interlocutors and suggests that this is an important consideration in matching of client and professional such as social worker or counsellor, a problematic area in child protection (Farmer and Owen 1995).

The model for black identity development cited in Robinson (1998) consists of developmental or adaptive stages ranging from 'conformity' when one devalues one's own group in preference to white standards, through stages of 'dissonance' where individuals are confused and ambivalent about their commitment to their own ethnic group; 'immersion–emersion' where individuals idealize their own group and denigrate that which is perceived as white, to 'internalization' and 'integrative awareness' where individuals express a positive self and group identity.

The model for white identity development, again cited in Robinson (1998), evolves through stages from limited knowledge of black people and a strong adherence to stereotypes, through confusion, conflict and contact avoidance, intolerance and racism to a better understanding of one's 'whiteness' without reference to racism and, with perseverance, to a final stage where individuals value inter-ethnic experience.

Ethnic matching

Many service providers assume that a black worker will be a better therapeutic match for black client than a white worker. Such an assumption seems questionable, if, for example, a black worker and black client are at different stages of self-identity (Robinson 1998). There are examples of client–worker difficulties when ethnic matching was 'crudely made and was more apparent than real' (Farmer and Owen 1995). The ethnic self-identity models may therefore serve as a useful tool in understanding relationships between black and white service providers and their black clients. But more research is needed. Moreover, there is a danger that such models could be 'corrupted into lazy psychological reductionism' (Robinson 1998), with the adherence to the very stereotypes that we have sought to avoid. Health professionals should not react negatively if a black client withdraws from intervention with a black or white worker but consider alternatives such as joint working so that the client is exposed to a positive black-white role model.

External processes

An individual's ability to adapt to cultural change and continuity is affected by many external processes that may slow down or arrest development of ethnic identity. Whites are socialized to avoid dealing with their own whiteness and to accept their own ethnocentric value biases and notions of white supremacy that operate on an individual, institutional and cultural level. Black people experience different realities, the most corrosive being racism and discrimination. They also have to contend with material poverty, inequalities in housing, access to health services and employment, social isolation and the stress of cultural dissonance, marginalization and barriers to communication. Class and gender differences operate within some ethnic groups. Black children are exposed to different socialization systems. Many children are reared in a 'dual system' of public (e.g. informal and formal education systems, media and literature) and private cultures based on cultural heritage (Roer-Strier 2001). Misunderstandings and conflicts arise between parents and agents of the host culture such as health visitors and social workers.

Health professionals need to acknowledge these different realities within ethnic groups and how they could lead to child abuse and neglect. Roer-Strier (2001) offers detailed recommendations for primary prevention. These include the development of a respectful curiosity about ethnic groups within a locality, recognition of the 'cultural logic' of child rearing practices and a non-judgemental attitude towards them, a celebration and promotion of positive practices throughout the community, and the use of alternative community support systems such as community parents or link workers to overcome conflict and confusion.

There are many sources of risk to children from ethnic groups living in such situations of stress, conflict and misunderstanding, but are they more likely to be abused?

Child abuse and neglect

Demography

Large population-based studies of child abuse and neglect conducted in the USA and cited in Ards, Chung and Myers (1998) have revealed an over-representation of African-American children, especially for infant homicide. This finding was invariably associated with poverty, male unemployment (Gillham et al. 1998) and the absence of social support (Korbin et al. 1998; Spearly and Lauderdale 1983). A notable exception has been the National Incidence Study (NIS), which revealed no ethnic disproportionality in the incidence of cases referred by agencies for investigation (Ards et al. 2001). This discrepancy has been attributed to sample selection and case substantiation bias and, more importantly, to apparent 'racial bias' in reporting suspect cases (Sedlak et al. 2001).

There have been no comparable population-based studies in the UK, but smaller studies again show that black children are over-represented in referrals to local authorities (Brandon et al. 1999). African-Caribbean children were more likely to be referred for suspected physical abuse and were less likely to be referred for sexual abuse, emotional abuse or neglect than white children. 'Asian' children were more likely to be referred for neglect (Barn et al. 1997).

The apparent ethnic disparities in the incidence of child abuse and neglect may be due to differing judgements concerning the threshold criteria for referral. Thus, child abuse reporting may be influenced by definitions of abuse that are avowedly culturally sensitive rather than being intrinsic to the act or outcome (Levinson et al. 1984).

It is important to establish a definition of child abuse that can be applied across cultural and ethnic boundaries.

Towards a definition

No cultural or ethnic group specifically endorses child abuse. However, situations may arise within a certain cultural group that may give rise to concern. Failure to allow for a cultural perspective in defining abuse promotes an ethnocentric position, whereas adopting a stance of false cultural relativism in which all judgements are suspended in the name of cultural rights could expose children to risk (Korbin 1991). Korbin has described a framework for formulating culturally appropriate definitions of child abuse using the following three levels:

1 Cultural differences in child rearing practices and beliefs, arguably the most problematic area, where cultural conflict is most likely;

2 Idiosyncratic departure from one's own cultural continuum of acceptable behaviour, a level at which child abuse is most legitimately defined across cultural contexts; and

3 Societal harm to children due to social and material impoverishment. *Physical punishment* of children is a case in point, present at three levels and pervasive across cultures as a child rearing practice.

Physical punishment

Physical punishment has been defined as 'physical force with the intention of causing the child to experience pain but not injury, for the purposes of correction or control of the child's behaviour' (Elliman and Lynch 2000).

It is widespread across all ethnic groups and socio-economic strata. However, in a national representative sample of 1000 parents in the US, Dietz (2000) found an increase in frequency and severity of physical punishment among African-Americans compared with white, Hispanic or Native Americans. Severe physical punishment was defined as shaking a child (2+ years), hitting a child with a hard object, slapping a child on the face, head or ears and pinching, compared with 'ordinary' punishment such as spanking or slapping a child on the hand, arm or leg. The greater reliance on physical punishment of children among Africans, African-Americans and African-Caribbeans has been a topic of considerable debate (Payne 1989; Dietz 2000). Some have sought cultural explanations (level 1), including the violence of slavery, colonialism and the African diaspora and the erosion of more traditional guards against culturally unacceptable behaviour that was provided by relatives and other adults. Others have posited societal explanations (level 3) such as overwhelming poverty and discrimination. Coser, cited in Dietz (2000), argues that these conditions create a climate of violence which then becomes socialized as part of the culture itself.

At the first level, the more severe forms of physical punishment could be regarded, by childcare professionals at least, as potentially abusive acts. In a south-east London borough, for example, 91 (10%) referrals to the child protection facility during the

5 year period (1985–1990) were children of West African parents with physical injuries: 14 were considered to be due to abuse and 46 the result of physical chastisement (Koromoa, personal communication). Given the cultural explanations, is it legitimate to make such a distinction?

A distinction can be attempted on the basis of *significant harm* done to the child, a notion firmly established in UK child care legislation (Children Act 1989). Harm is defined as ill-treatment or impaired health and development which is attributable to the care given to the child (Section 31.2). Significance results from a comparison with the health and development that could reasonably be expected of a similar child (Section 31.10). In forming a judgement, professionals are required to give 'due consideration' to the child's cultural, linguistic and religious background (Section 22.5). This clause provides a legal framework for anti-racist practice and should not be regarded as an invitation to indulge in false cultural relativism and the use of cultural stereotypes. Unless one takes the view that all physical punishment is abusive, a judgement still has to be reached.

Finklehor and Korbin (1988) have proposed a definition of abuse in which the harm is *proscribed*, i.e., the action that caused the harm is 'negatively valued' by dint of its deviance, its violation of legal codes or social expectations and its harmful intent. The dimension of *intentionality* is very important when attempting to estimate harm. For example, when a mother burns a child's fingers for stealing, the harm is very intentional, compared with (arguably) a 'spanking' on the bottom. The *severity* of both the action and its consequences for the child is also important. A number of studies of various cultural groups suggest an intracultural consensus (level 2) on what is viewed as abuse when the action is deemed intentional and when the consequences are severe (Collier *et al.* 1999; Lau *et al.* 1999; Elliot *et al.* 1997; Payne 1989). In Barbados, for example, there was a consensus, especially among the young, that lashing out, burning or scalding, prolonged flogging causing marks and public chastisement were acts intended to cause harm and that such acts may have an adverse outcome for the children, promoting poor self-esteem and engendering an aggression and hostility. Authors such as Strauss (2000) and Elliman and Lynch (2000) also emphasize the negative long-term consequences of physical punishment, including its escalation to physical abuse. They argue for a general consensus against all forms of physical punishment of children, despite evident societal and legislative sanction in most countries, with the notable exception of Sweden.

There is, argue Finklehor and Kolvin (1988), an emerging consensus that can challenge local norms, and the acceptance that demonstrable serious physical and mental harm may occasion some forms of physical punishment is certainly one component. This can give rise to a more constructive community approach to the exploration of alternative strategies for child rearing without recourse to physical punishment and which regard family violence as unacceptable (Eisenberg 1981). Such an approach will only succeed in preventing child abuse if the processes that disadvantage black children are addressed.

An international consensus on common rights that apply to children has now been agreed. Born out of a belief in the existence of 'common values' necessary to resolve cultural disputes, it is capable of a strong moral stand against child abuse and exploitation.

The UN Convention on the Rights of the Child

The UN Convention on the Rights of the Child (1989) was unanimously adopted by the UN General Assembly in 1989 and has since been ratified by every government, with the notable exception of the USA and Somalia (which has no government). It came into force in Britain in 1992. It sets universally appropriate and humane obligations towards children and sets standards for the protection of children against neglect, abuse, exploitation, and discrimination (Articles 3, 6, 19, 32, 34 and 36). It also implores us to listen to the voice of the child (Article 12). The Convention therefore represents a strong international consensus and provides professionals and other advocates with a tool to protect children from apparent excesses of local custom, practice and legal systems (Munir 1993). Female genital mutilation is an example. The British Association for Community Child Health (BACCH) has published a useful practitioners' guide to the implementation of the UN Convention within the National Health Service (Child Health Rights).

Female genital mutilation

The ancient practice of female genital mutilation occurs across sub-Saharan Africa, extending in East Africa from Egypt in the north to Tanzania in the south. It is also found in parts of the Arabian and Malay peninsulas. It crosses cultural and religious boundaries but survives in situations of patriachy and social control of women (Barstow 1999; Black and Debelle 1995). With the exception of Egypt, the geographical distribution of the practice corresponds to countries that share great poverty, lack of basic amenities such as running water, and very high infant mortality rates. There are three variations of mutilation, of which the most severe, infibulation, involves cutting off all of the external genitalia and sewing up the wound leaving only a pinhole meatus. Numerous rationales and justifications for this practice have been posited. Useful, detailed, well-referenced and wide-ranging discussions of this subject can be found in Barstow (1999), Black and Debelle (1995), Webb and Hartley (1994) and McLean and Graham (1985).

Female genital mutilation is worthy of discussion, if only to recognize that it exists in multicultural societies including the UK and that it can provide a model for good practice that combines child protection with community education and advocacy at local, national and international level. It is estimated that in the UK 10,000 girls are at risk of genital mutilation, (Webb and Hartley 1994). Surveys of obstetricians and midwives suggest that the practice is widespread among Somali and Yemenis (Lawrence, personal communication). It represents a dilemma in child protection in that the practice is perceived as a *responsible act* by parents to ensure their daughter a place in society, yet is an illegal practice. It is not done with an intention to harm yet the consequences are severe for the child, both physically and psychologically. What kind of approach is appropriate when one discovers that a girl has been, or is at risk of being, mutilated?

Local inter-agency child protection procedures may dictate that a referral to a statutory agency is undertaken. This will allow a detailed, sensitive and non-judgemental assessment of the child to be undertaken, in which the meaning of mutilation is considered in relation to other interrelated contexts of meaning such as the child herself and her stories, family narratives and the social and cultural mores. This should be undertaken using appropriate interpreters and community members. If a child has been mutilated, a police investigation will also be undertaken. Webb and Hartley (1994) state that 'female genital mutilation will only be eradicated by the communities themselves, whether resident in Africa or elsewhere'. Eradication should be an exchange for 'an overall strategy to improve the health and social welfare of the population as a whole' and to support the cultural fabric. Thus, advocacy at all levels is crucial. For example, one must be prepared to support the work of organizations such as the Foundation for Women's Health, Research and Development (FORWARD) who actively engage with and support women who remain attached to their own cultural heritage but who are prepared to call into question traditional practices that endanger their lives and health. At a local level, education initiatives must be coupled with other initiatives such as 'well woman clinics', staffed by specialist midwives and community parents or peer counsellors.

Folk remedies and child abuse

Most authorities agree that the cutaneous lesions left by certain folk remedies should not be taken as potentially abusive. Health professionals should be familiar with any practices being maintained by ethnic groups within their locality because of the potential confusion with child abuse. These remedies have been extensively reviewed by Hansen (1997) and include coining (or *cao gio*), a South-east Asian folk remedy to ameliorate a variety of symptoms. The symptomatic area is massaged with medicated oil and then rubbed in a downward linear fashion with the edge of a coin or other object until bruising occurs. An example of the marks left is shown in Fig. 4.1.

Pinching is a related practice. Lesions from therapeutic burning (maquas) or cupping may also be seen but are relatively rare.

A more common source of confusion and referral to child protection services are the ubiquitous 'mongolian blue spots'. These are blue discolourations, present from birth and seen on the lower back, and occasionally on the arms and legs of infants from most ethnic groups. Familiar to parents, they may be mistaken for bruises to a child's back by other carers such as day care staff, especially if the spots are large and extensive (Dungy 1982). This can be avoided by education of staff and by having the spots documented in the child's personal health record.

Conclusion

The recognition of child abuse in a multicultural context should be considered in the light of a knowledge and understanding of local cultural and ethnic beliefs, customs and practices. Such knowledge can be gained through education and training and, more importantly, through the development of respectful curiosity. The test of 'significant harm' should be applied to any case of suspected abuse, taking into account such factors as intent to harm, severity, in terms of both the action and the outcome,

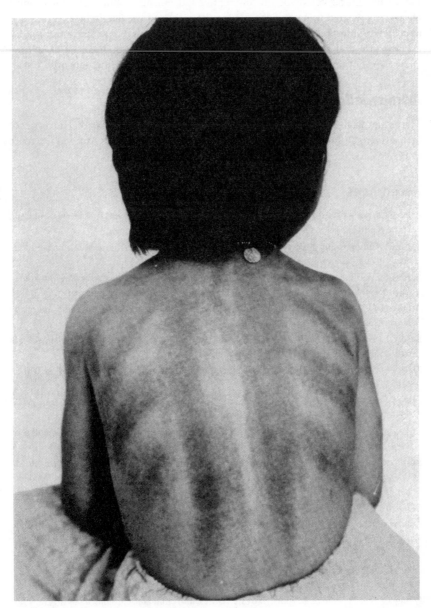

Figure 4.1 Symmetrical pupura caused by coin-rubbing.

and how much it violates the child's right to dignity and protection, as judged by absolute standards such as the UN Convention. It is very important to guard against the use of cultural stereotypes in coming to a judgement. Health professionals must always be prepared to be an advocate for the child and the family by ensuring that appropriate interpreters and community supports are used and that interventions acknowledge and are sensitive to the stress engendered by the realities of cultural change and continuity, racism, discrimination, marginalization, and poverty.

Acknowledgements

The author would like to thank Mr Ash Chand, Centre for Social Work, University of Nottingham, Dr John Koramoa, St Giles Hospital, London and Ms Amanda Lawrence of FORWARD for permission to use their data.

References

Ards SD, Chung C and Myers SL (2001) Sample selection bias and racial differences in child abuse reporting: once again. *Child Abuse and Neglect* 25: 7–12.

Ards SD, Chung C and Myers SL (1998) The effects of sample selection bias on racial differences in child abuse reporting. *Child Abuse and Neglect* 22: 103–15.

Barn R, Sinclair R and Ferdinand D (1997) *Acting on Principle: an Examination of Race and Ethnicity in Social Services Provision for Children and Families.* London: BAAF.

Barstow DG (1999) Female genital mutilation: the penultimate gender abuse. *Child Abuse and Neglect* 23: 501–10.

Belsky J (1980) Child maltreatment: an ecological integration. *American Psychologist* 35: 320–35.

Black JA and Debelle GD (1995) Female genital mutilation in Britain. *British Medical Journal* 310: 1590–92.

Brah A (1994) Time, place, and others: discourses of race, nation, and ethnicity. *Sociology* 28: 805–13.

Brandon M, Thorn J, Lewes A and Way A (1999) *Safeguarding Children with the Children Act 1989.* London: HMSO.

Burnham J and Harris Q (1996) Emerging ethnicity. A tale of three cultures, in K. Dwivedi and U Varma (eds) *Meeting the Needs of Ethnic Minority Children: a Handbook for Professionals.* London: Jessica Kingsley.

Children Act 1989 (1989) London: HMSO.

Collier AF, McClure FH, Collier J, Otto C and Polloi A (1999) Culture-specific views of child maltreatment and parenting styles in a Pacific-Island community. *Child Abuse and Neglect* 23: 229–44.

Dietz TL (2000) Disciplining children: characteristics associated with the use of corporal punishment. *Child Abuse and Neglect* 24: 1529–42.

Dungy CI (1982) Mongolian spots, day care centres, and child abuse. *Pediatrics* 69: 672.

Eisenberg L (1981) Cross-cultural and historical perspectives on child abuse and neglect. *Child Abuse and Neglect* 5: 299–308.

Elliman D and Lynch MA (2000) The physical punishment of children. *Archives of Disease in Childhood* 83: 196–8.

Elliott JM, Tong CK and Tan PM (1997) Attitudes of the Singapore public to actions suggesting child abuse. *Child Abuse and Neglect* 21: 445–64.

Farmer E and Owen M (1995) *Child Protection Practice: Private Risks and Public Remedies.* London: HMSO.

Finkelhor D and Korbin J (1988) Child abuse as an international issue. *Child Abuse and Neglect* 12: 3–23.

Garbarino J (1977) The human ecology of maltreatment: A conceptual model for research. *Journal of Marriage and the Family* 39: 721–35.

Gillham B, Tanner G, Cheyne B, Freeman I, Rooney M and Lambie A (1998) Unemployment rates, single parent density, and indices of child poverty: Their relationship to different categories of child abuse and neglect. *Child Abuse and Neglect* 22: 79–90.

Hansen KK (1997) Folk remedies and child abuse: a review with emphasis on caida de mollera and its relationship to shaken baby syndrome. *Child Abuse and Neglect* 22: 117–27.

Hillier S and Kelleher D (1996) Considering culture, ethnicity and the politics of health, in D Kelleher, S Hillier (eds) *Researching Cultural Differences in Health.* London: Routledge.

Howze DC and Kotch JB (1984) Disentangling life events, stress, and social support: implications for the primary prevention of child abuse and neglect. *Child Abuse and Neglect* 8: 401–9.

Kelleher D (1996) A defence of the use of the terms 'ethnicity' and 'culture', in D Kelleher, S Hillier (eds) *Researching Cultural Differences in Health.* London: Routledge.

Korbin JE, Coulton CJ, Chard S, Platt-Houston C and Su M (1998) Impoverishment and child, maltreatment in African American and European American neighbourhoods. *Development and Psychology* 10: 215–33.

Korbin JE (1991) Cross-cultural perspectives and research directions for the 21st century. *Child Abuse and Neglect* 15(suppl 1): 67–77.

Lau JTF, Liu JLY, Yu A and Wong CK (1999) Conceptualization, reporting and underreporting of child abuse in Hong Kong. *Child Abuse and Neglect* 23: 1159–74.

Levinson RM and Graves WL (1984) Cross-cultural variations in the definition of child abuse: nurses in the United States and the United Kingdom. *Child Abuse and Neglect* 21: 35–44.

McLean S and Graham SE (1985) *Female Circumcision, Excision and Infibulation.* The Minority Rights Group, Report No. 47. London: Minority Rights Group.

Munir ABB (1993) Child protection: principles and applications. *Child Abuse Review* 2: 119–26.

Parekh P (2000) *Rethinking Multiculturalism.* London: Macmillan.

Payne MA (1989) Use and abuse of corporal punishment: a Caribbean view. *Child Abuse and Neglect* 13: 389–401.

Pfeffer N (1998) Theories of race, ethnicity and culture. *British Medical Journal* 317: 1381–4.

Robinson L (1998) *'Race', Communication and the Caring Professions.* Buckingham: Open University Press.

Roer-Strier D (2001) Reducing risk for children in changing cultural contexts: recommendations for intervention and training. *Child Abuse and Neglect* 25: 23148.

Sedlak AJ, Bruce C and Schultz DJ (2001) Letter to the editor. *Child Abuse and Neglect* 25: 1–5.

Senior PA and Bhopal R (1994) Ethnicity as a variable in epidemiological research. *British Medical Journal* 309: 327–30.

Smaje C (1995) *Health, Race and Ethnicity.* London: Kings Fund.

Spearly JL and Lauderdale M (1983) Community characteristics and ethnicity in the prediction of child maltreatment rates. *Child Abuse and Neglect* 7: 91–105.

Strauss MA (2000) Corporal punishment and primary prevention of physical abuse. *Child Abuse and Neglect* 24: 1109–14.

Strauss MM (1980) Stress and physical child abuse. *Child Abuse and Neglect* 4: 75–88.

United Nations General Assembly (1989) *Adoption of a Convention on the Rights of the Child.* UN Document A/Res/44/25.

Webb E and Hartley B (1994) Female genital mutilation: a dilemma in child protection. *Archives of Disease in Childhood* 70: 441–4.

Wilson-Oyelaran EB (1989) The ecological model and the study of child abuse in Nigeria. *Child Abuse and Neglect* 13: 379–87.

Chapter 5

The training needs care of primary health teams in child protection

Michael J. Bannon, Yvonne H. Carter,
Neil R. Jackson and Mitch Blair

Introduction

The child protection framework in England is defined within *Working Together to Safeguard Children* (Department of Health 1999). This document, a substantial revision of previous versions, clearly defines both the roles and responsibilities of all health professionals in the overall process of ensuring that children are protected from the threat of abuse or neglect (cf. Table 5.1). Successful implementation of child protection procedures is, in part therefore, dependent on appropriate responsive behaviour on the part of all professionals who maintain significant contact with children and their families. Health care workers are required to maintain constant

Table 5.1 The involvement of health professionals in work with children and families

The involvement of health professionals is important at all stages of work with children and families
◆ Recognizing children in need of support and/or safeguarding, and parents who may need extra help in bringing up their children;
◆ Contributing to enquiries about a child and family;
◆ Assessing the needs of children and the capacity of parents to meet their children's needs;
◆ Planning and providing support to vulnerable children and families;
◆ Participating in child protection conferences;
◆ Planning support for children at risk of significant harm;
◆ Providing therapeutic help to abused children and parents under stress (e.g. mental illness);
◆ Playing a part, through the child protection plan, in safeguarding children from significant harm; and contributing to case reviews.
There will always be a need for close cooperation with other agencies, including any other health professionals involved.

From Department of Health (1999).

Table 5.2 Stages in the child protection process with resulting requirements in knowledge, skills and attitudes

Stage	Knowledge	Skills	Attitudes
Recognition of abuse	Predisposing factors Clinical indicators	Clinical acumen Developmental examination	Acceptance that abuse is prevalent
Reporting	Local reporting arrangements Role appreciation When to intervene	Interviewing skills Documentation	Acceptance of paramountcy principle Acknowledgement of adverse effects of abuse and neglect
Investigation	Role appreciation Role of others	Communication skills Report writing	Willingness to share information Co-operation with other agencies Coping skills

vigilance for the possibility of abuse or neglect and to report their concerns or suspicions as appropriate to the statutory agencies. They are then expected to participate in subsequent inter-agency investigations and intervention.

The child protection process might be considered to consist of several sequential steps or stages, each of which has training and educational implications for health professionals (Table 5.2). Child protection training is now universally acknowledged to represent an integral component of the overall process of ensuring that children remain safe from the threat of maltreatment by their carers. In some parts of the world, such is the perceived importance of training, that active participation by professionals of all relevant disciplines is compulsory (Reiniger *et al.* 1995). In England considerable efforts have already been undertaken by training subcommittees of Area Child Protection Committees (ACPCs) in order to ensure that multi-professional training is readily available to all. Participation in training events in England, however, is voluntary.

In this chapter we will consider:

1 Why child protection training is essential for primary health care professionals;

2 How primary care specific child protection training might be developed;

3 Examples of innovative child protection training for primary care.

Training for clinical staff in the identification and management of child abuse and neglect is now considered to represent an appropriate use of resources for several reasons.

Child abuse work is demanding

There is universal agreement with respect to the challenging nature of child abuse work. The ultimate in clinical acumen, decision-making ability and communication skills are required. Abuse or neglect may present in a myriad of confusing and deceptive ways that may result in delayed detection. Unlike other clinical situations, diagnosis of child abuse with a high degree of certainty is not always possible. Furthermore, many professionals find it intimidating to confront parents and carers.

Others have deep-rooted reservations about sharing sensitive information with outside agencies. In order for professionals to successfully undertake their responsibility in the child protection process, they must be sure of their own role and responsibility in this respect, possess sufficient confidence to challenge suspicions related to clinical presentations and know what to do and who to inform. Furthermore they must be equipped with the coping strategies necessary in order to deal with the complex emotions evoked by child abuse cases.

Professionals have inadequate knowledge of child abuse and neglect

Working Together outlines the demands placed upon health professionals in terms of child protection knowledge and skills. They must fully appreciate the circumstances likely to result in child maltreatment and also recognize clinical indicators of abuse or neglect. It is essential that they acknowledge that child abuse exists, that it is prevalent and has adverse effects on child welfare. They must also understand their own role and that of others in the overall child protection process.

Clinical staff, both doctors and nurses, when surveyed have demonstrated impaired awareness of child protection issues and have on occasion expressed dissatisfaction both with their levels of knowledge and extent of training. For example, continuing deficiencies in knowledge and awareness of child sexual abuse over a ten year period were found among doctors in Ohio (Lentsch and Johnson 2000). The inadequate knowledge of Israeli doctors of physical abuse has also been documented (Offer-Shechter *et al.* 2000). Paediatric emergency trainees in North America were unhappy with both the amount and quality of their child protection training (Wright *et al.* 1999). Similar perceptions were found among GP registrars in North London (Bannon *et al.* 2001).

Little is currently known of the training needs of other professional members of the primary health care team (PCHT), with the exception of health visitors. Health visitors in the UK undertake a substantial front line role in child protection work. Their knowledge and training is widely perceived to be superior to other community nurses who work with children and their families. Their role, mode of working and training in this area has been critically reviewed (Ling and Luker 2000). However, at least one study in South London has revealed that health visitors felt their initial training in child protection was less than adequate (Gilardi 1991). At present, little has been published regarding the child protection training of other members of the PCHT and this might represent a priority for future educational research.

Health professionals frequently fail to recognize and report abuse

Although the media may occasionally suggest that health professionals, particularly doctors, demonstrate a tendency to be overzealous in their accusations of abuse, the reality is more likely to be one of under recognition and inefficient reporting. Child protection experts in both the USA and UK have repeatedly expressed concern at the inability of doctors of all grades of seniority and disciplines to recognize serious instances of abuse, even when highly indicative clues were present. A UK review of subdural haematomas in infants resulting from intentional injury demonstrated that in a significant number of cases, appropriate suspicion was not raised and the diagnosis of abuse was not made (Jayawant *et al.* 1998). Similar findings were evident from a comparable survey in the USA (Leventhal 1999).

Attitudes held by health professionals may influence their reporting behaviour

Research has shown that personal attributes of clinicians, along with their beliefs and attitudes, may profoundly influence their responsiveness and reporting behaviour when confronted with suspected child abuse. A significant minority of doctors in Queensland would not report suspected child abuse to the statutory agencies despite a legal mandate to do so (Van Haeringen *et al.* 1998). The reasons given were multiple but revolved around a perceived lack of confidence in Social Services. Israeli paediatricians were more likely to diagnose abuse if the presenting evidence was concrete and biased toward biomedical issues (Shor 1998). This suggested impaired awareness of relevant psychosocial issues. It would appear that attitudes held by doctors in this respect are formed early. English medical students had already similar perceptions regarding diagnosis and reporting of abuse when compared to those of qualified doctors (Warner-Rodgers *et al.* 1996).

There is now some evidence that training programmes can produce measurable improvements in the knowledge, skills and attitudes of professionals in the area of child protection. Much of this work has been undertaken with those who are most likely to be exposed to child abuse situations – teachers, social workers and police – and much can be learned from this experience for application to primary health care worker training. In one randomized trial of a one day training of teachers, the experimental group were significantly more likely to talk with individual students to determine if the abuse was occurring, were more likely to give a class presentation on child abuse, were less likely to report the use of physical punishment in the classroom and more likely to discuss child abuse with colleagues (Hazzard and Rupp 1983).

In addition there is now some research to suggest that child protection training will positively influence the attitudes of doctors toward participation in the child protection process. One study encouragingly found a positive correlation between reporting behaviour and the amount of child protection training received among US military physicians (Lawrence and Brannen 2000).

General Practitioners and child protection

Primary health care professionals play an important role in the delivery of health to children throughout the world. In the UK, they undertake an enhanced responsibility in this respect. In the first instance, GPs, rather than paediatricians, are usually the first point of contact for the majority of childhood illness which require a professional opinion. In addition, they now undertake the majority of child health promotion and surveillance activities. As a result, they have continuous, frequent and unique contact with children and their families. Acknowledging the high prevalence of child maltreatment, it seems inevitable that members of the primary heath care team (PHCT) will continually encounter children in need of protection.

GPs therefore have much to offer to the child protection process. However, they have been the subject of criticism regarding their performance in the child protection process upon three accounts:

1 Experience reveals that despite having contact with children known to be at risk, they, of all of the professional groups, were least likely to invoke child protection procedures (Hallett and Birchall 1994).

2 Social workers have frequently commented on the apparent infrequent attendance of GPs at child protection case conferences (Simpson *et al.* 1994).[1]

3 Several surveys have shown that of the many professional groups involved in the care of children, GPs have received the least amount of child protection training (Hendry 1997). In addition, child protection trainers have complained that having undertaken training needs analysis, there was subsequently poor attendance by GPs at specially organized child protection training events. These findings are not limited to the UK. A survey among Irish GPs revealed similar behaviour (Payne 1999).

Child abuse presents the GP with particular difficulties that result from the inherent tensions arising from conflict between the philosophies of child protection and that of primary care (Figure 5.1). Many GPs, while respecting the basic notion that the safety of children must be paramount, admit to ambivalent feelings about the validity of child protection procedures in general (Carter 1995).

The implications from these factors are that in the first instance training is required in order to increase GPs' awareness of abuse and neglect, and that educational initiatives are also needed in order to effect appropriate attitudinal change.

Primary care	Child protection
Focused on provision of care for families	Focused upon welfare of the child primarily
Confidentiality is a guiding principle	Information sharing is essential
Professional autonomy is a strong tradition i.e. GPs are independent providers of health care	Interagency collaboration is fundamental to child protection process

Figure 5.1 Primary care and child protection – inherent tensions of two models of care.

[1] See also Chapter 15.

A suggested framework for meeting the child protection training needs of primary health care teams

In order that child protection training for primary health care teams is successful in its objectives of ensuring the safety of children, it is essential that it is implemented in a manner that adheres to agreed principles of adult learning and curriculum development as follows:

1 There should be clarity with respect to the aims and objectives of training;

2 There must be agreement with respect to the most appropriate content of training;

3 It should be delivered in an acceptable form and at the most appropriate time to the target audience;

4 The impact of any new training initiatives must be evaluated according to agreed criteria and appropriate changes made.

Aims and objectives of child protection training

In many respects, *Working Together* provides clear guidance with respect to the aims and objectives of child protection training for all professionals. Specific objectives for the PCHT should therefore include the following:

1 All members of the PHCT should embrace the philosophy of the child paramountcy principle.[2]

2 They should appreciate their own role and that of others (both within and outside of the PCHT) in the child protection process.

3 An adequate knowledge of the precursors of child maltreatment, including its clinical indicators, should represent part of their core knowledge.

4 They must know precisely what is expected of then when they suspect abuse or neglect in terms of what to do and say.

Child protection curriculum development

In order to define the most appropriate training curriculum for the PHCT there must be a compromise between the following:

1 Standards of knowledge and competencies as directed by professional bodies and by government statute. These will vary between individual countries; in England guidance is provided by *Working Together* (Departement of Health 1999);

2 Views of child protection training experts regarding the scope and content of training;

3 Perceptions of the potential trainees, in this case GPs and other members of the PHCT.

....

[2] i.e. the safety and welfare of the child is *paramount* and overrides all other considerations.

Definition of training needs

Two workshops were held by one of the authors (MB) with the National Society for the Prevention of Cruelty to Children (NSPCC) trainers in Birmingham 1998 in order to define the most pertinent child protection training themes for GPs and other members of the PHCT. A combination of closed and open questions were used in order to focus upon training themes. The following, after discussion, were considered to represent the most important topics in order of priority:

1 Appreciation of the importance of interagency working and teamwork in child protection

2 Awareness of the clinical indicators of abuse and neglect within the setting of primary care

3 Recognition that one's own personal attitudes towards this subject might profoundly influence clinical behaviour

4 Knowledge of the child protection process in general as well as local procedures

5 Basic understanding of the legal framework currently in place for the protection of children.

While acknowledging the experience and opinions of child protection training experts, the views of the target audience regarding the content of child protection training must not be overlooked. Research has already confirmed that school teachers have unmet and previously unrecognized training needs which reflected upon their unique role with children and their carers (Braun 1993). We believed that GPs and other members of the PHCT also had unmet training needs in this respect. A first step in curriculum development should therefore be a thorough training needs analysis that was undertaken by the authors (MB and YHC) in three stages:

1 Review of published literature

2 Focus group discussions among five PCHTs in the West Midlands

3 Questionnaire survey among GPs in England in 1996.

Conclusions from this combined exercise were as follows.

Literature review

We could find no single paper published up to 1996 that adequately addressed the issues associated with meeting the training needs of GPs and other members of the PCHT. However, a number of useful themes were evident, all of which had implications for child protection training.

♦ In some countries child abuse is considered to represent part of a wider spectrum of domestic violence that includes spouse and elder abuse. Training programmes have been widened in focus to reflect this broader focus (Tildern et al. 1994).

♦ Doctors of all backgrounds, including those who work in primary care, demonstrate a reluctance to report instances of suspected abuse, even in countries where such reporting is mandatory (Van Haeringen et al. 1998).

◆ Personal characteristics of doctors (i.e. age, sex, personal history of abuse, previous training on child protection) influence their behaviour when they encounter instances of suspected child abuse (Johnson 1993).

◆ The legal, moral and ethical dimensions of the GP's role in child protection work are also worthy of consideration. Confidentiality remains a powerful medical tradition and many doctors have reservations about sharing sensitive information with statutory agencies. At the same time, others are fearful of the repercussions of not reporting instances of abuse (van Veenendaal 1993).

Focus group discussions

Five focus group discussions, consisting of 38 participants, 16 of whom were GPs, were held in a variety of settings within the West Midlands in order to allow GPs to discuss issues relevant to their involvement in child protection work with other members of the primary health care team. It was found that there was considerable confusion with respect to a precise definition of the role of the GP in child protection work; this confusion was expressed both by the GPs themselves and by other members of the PHCT.

Child protection was a source of considerable anxiety and uncertainty to GPs. This was especially the case with respect to definition of their role in child protection work, their lack of clarity with respect to referral processes and the potential for damage to their relationship with families when they initiated child protection procedures.

GPs held ambivalent views with respect to their attendance at child protection case conferences, with many expressing the opinion that they had little to contribute to the process.

Of all of the professional groups represented, GPs had received the least amount of child protection training. However, all GPs felt that more training on this subject was needed.

Questionnaire survey

A postal, confidential questionnaire survey which attempted to determine GP child protection training needs by means of open and closed questions received 1,000 responses from GPs working in England. The main training themes elicited were:

◆ Detection of abuse:
the need to develop improved standards in the prompt identification of all types of child abuse and neglect as well as alertness to the clinical indicators of abuse.

◆ Legal aspects:
improved understanding of recent legislation
an appreciation of the medico–legal implications for doctors of their involvement in the child protection process.

◆ Intervention procedures once abuse was suspected:
appreciation of when the threshold for intervention had been exceeded;
local referral processes.

- Inter-agency liaison:
  appreciation of the roles of other agencies in the child protection process (Social Services, Police, Accident and Emergency Departments);
  means of communicating with them.

- Child protection case conferences:
  a greater understanding of the wider implications for them when they attended conferences; guidance with respect to the preparation and presentation of reports for conferences; how to deal with the presence of parents at conferences.

Personal characteristics of respondents had profound influences upon their perceptions in this respect, with different training priorities identified by those GPs who were female, more experienced, and those who had qualified overseas.

Curriculum development

The next task was concerned with the development of a new training package that would be sensitive to the main issues identified within the various training needs analysis exercises. An informal steering group was formed with representation from the authors, the NSPCC and the General Practice Department of the (then) North Thames Postgraduate Deanery. Following appropriate discussion it was agreed to target the training needs of GPs while they were in training (referred to as GP registrars). The perceived advantages of this approach were in the first instance that GP registrars could be regarded as a captive audience amenable to training, as efforts to engage established GPs have to date been less than successful. Furthermore it was argued that if training on this topic was successfully implemented during a formative phase of their vocational education, then positive attitudes toward child protection issues might be formed with future benefit.

Prior to the implementation of the newly developed training package, a further training needs analysis consisting of a postal questionnaire was sent to all GP registrars in North Thames, 112 (74%) of whom responded. It was found that that, overall, registrars had received some training on more general aspects of child abuse and neglect including its predisposing factors and presenting features. Aspects of child protection work, which could be considered to be more specific to primary care, were not covered in training and hence were seen as unmet training needs. The main themes for future child protection training included:

- What to do and say when abuse was suspected during the course of a consultation
- Awareness of local child protection guidelines and strategies for their implementation at practice level
- How to maintain working relationships with families during and after the child abuse investigative process
- Attendance at child protection case conferences and preparation of relevant reports.

Registrars who qualified outside of the UK had received less undergraduate child protection training compared to UK graduates. Female registrars rated several topics as being more relevant for future training when compared with their male colleagues.

It was disappointing to find that 46 registrars (41%) had received no postgraduate training on the topic while 44 (40%) had experienced theoretical training only. ('Theoretical training' consisted of lectures, tutorials and in some cases attendance at multidisciplinary Area Child Protection Committee seminars.) Twenty respondents (18%) had, in addition, some degree of practical child protection experience. This included supervised involvement in the assessment of suspected cases of child abuse; five registrars had attended one or more child protection case conferences, and one registrar gave evidence in a family court.

Respondents were critical of their postgraduate child protection training on two accounts. First, while generic, theoretical child abuse training was welcomed, it was not considered to be especially sensitive to primary care. Second, there was an expressed view that suitable training opportunities were being missed during vocational training in the sense that during their Senior House Officer attachments, GP registrars were bypassed when child protection cases came to the paediatric wards. There also appeared to be little involvement with this subject during their year in general practice either. Not surprisingly, only 27 respondents (24%) considered themselves to be adequately prepared for future child protection work.

The main themes identified from the various exercises were prioritized and existing training packages critically examined in order to identify relevant material that could be easily adopted for this purpose.

The aims and objectives of child protection for GP registrars were defined as the following:

On completion of the course it was hoped that participants would be able to:

1 Describe the legal context of child protection

2 Demonstrate an understanding of the definitions of abuse and threshold for action

3 Develop strategies for the management of child protection issues in general practice

4 Demonstrate skills in communicating child protection concerns to carers, children and professional agencies

5 Recognize and give value to the emotional impact of child protection work.

Training was delivered in two parts. Prior to a half-day workshop, each registrar was provided with written material and other background information. This consisted of concise summaries of the *Children Act 1989, Working Together* (Department of Health 1999) as well as primary care, specific child protection epidemiology and clinical presentations. Training materials previously developed by the NSPCC were specifically amended for this purpose.

The second part of the training package consisted of a half-day seminar, directed by MB and a Training Officer from the NSPCC. A highly interactive format was used. Thirty-one registrars (mean age 33 years, 20 were male and 19 had qualified in the UK) attended three workshops during the summer of 1999. The format is given in Table 5.3.

Evaluation of the training event revealed significant change in attitudes and levels of confidence in dealing with future child protection issues, at least in the short term. Overall participants welcomed the opportunity for training and found the session enjoyable.

Table 5.3 Format of training programme

Introductions: Hopes and fears Ground rules Aims and objectives	(20 mins)
Exercise: Signs, symptoms, definitions Thresholds Legal responsibilities	(30 mins) (10 mins)
Small group exercise: Inhibitors to disclosure Feedback Break	(40 mins) (15 mins)

Case study (consequences of action):

Family:
Mother: Maria, 22 years, unemployed
Father: Not known
Child: Patty aged 21 weeks

Maria has brought Patty to the surgery although she has made the appointment for herself because she is feeling run down. During the course of the consultation, Maria describes Patty as 'looking like a monkey' and complains that she is slow to learn and difficult to feed. Patty now weighs only 6lb 13oz; she was eight weeks premature and weighed 4lb 3oz at birth. The pregnancy was concealed and Maria had not booked for ante-natal care. Maria, prior to the pregnancy, was a student and gave birth a few weeks before the end of her course. Her extended family live in Spain and Maria has no friends in England.

1   What are the areas of concern?
2   What does this situation suggest to you?
3   What (if anything) should you do?

(40 mins)

Role play: Communicating concerns Feedback Developing a protocol for practice Evaluation	(50 mins) (20 mins) (15 mins)

Practice-based training

The preceding exercise represents an example of uni-professional training. We are now aware of the fact that many districts within the UK have attempted PCHT-orientated child protection training. This model is based on the premise that most principals in general practice already have some experiences of dealing with child abuse, and that training time is limited and needs to be tailored specifically to the practice team. It also assumes that those who require training most are not necessarily likely to seek it out actively, just because it is on offer as part of a wider postgraduate programme. Its aim is to target large numbers of GPs and community nurses with a view to engaging them in a non-threatening environment. One example of this type of training is now described below in detail (Polnay and Blair 1999).

Practitioners were directly approached by the trainers (a GP medical advisor for child protection and a Consultant Community Paediatrician) by telephone to ask if they would host the session in their practice and advertise it appropriately to staff. This gave the practitioner the responsibility of ensuring that the training had appropriate priority amongst so many other competing training priorities. The format in this programme consisted of a two hour practice-based interactive session with a 15 minute break. The session starts with an audiotape of an adult survivor, describing her experiences of being abused as a child, which was designed to highlight the need for early detection and prevention. Participants subsequently identified particular areas which they have found difficult around child protection and would like included in the session. There followed a lecture on the relevance of child protection to general practice, the framework of the local child protection committees and emphasis on the four key themes of recognition, communication, child protection procedures and record keeping. Slides were shown to illustrate clinical examples of physical, emotional, and sexual abuse and neglect in children of different ages with an emphasis on history taking and clinical examination skills. A set of case scenarios and participant discussions were used to highlight the need for meticulous observation and recording in clinical records. These scenarios also gave an opportunity for the rehearsal of 'scripts' to practice communication between practitioner and the carers, with other members of practice team as well as outside agencies. Practical information about referral formats and telephone contacts of key personnel was also given.

Within 13 months, 57% of all target practices in the District had received training of this style, the content and quality of which was highly evaluated. Although subsequent child abuse reporting behaviour of the participants was not measured, 98% stated that they were confident in their knowledge base for taking appropriate action in cases of suspected abuse. As described earlier, this is an area which others have cited as being deficient in their training.

Conclusions and areas for further work and consideration

◆ The need for effective and primary care sensitive training in child protection for GPs and other members of the PCHT is self-evident. PCHT members have specific and to date unmet training needs in this area and coordinated efforts are required in order to address these needs.

◆ There is a paucity of research around child protection and primary care. Little is known of the training needs of reception staff, practice nurses, therapists and other members of the PHCT who have frequent contact with children and their families.

This represents an area for further research. Furthermore, the collective training needs of the primary health care team require further evaluation.

◆ A variety of training modalities and opportunities are needed.

• There is a need for uni-professional child protection training that is directed specifically at members of a distinct professional group, such as health visitors or GP registrars.

• Multi-professional training is also required and is widely available from Area Child Protection Committees. This will emphasize multidisciplinary implications of child protection work.

• We believe that there is in addition a need for team-based training. Each PCHT is a discrete and unique organization with its own peculiarities in terms of patient need and skill mix of professionals. Learning together as a team should enhance appreciation of roles and mutual support and respect.

• Child protection training should be considered as a continuum beginnin in a professionals' pre-qualification years and being consolidated during their professional training. It follows that this subject should also be part of continuing professional development.

• The impact of child protection training must be evaluated in both the long and short term. Early outcome measures might include improvements in attitudes, knowledge and levels of confidence. However, the real test of the effectiveness of child protection training will be its impact on the behaviour of health professionals whenever they encounter a child in need of protection.

• The newly formed Primary Care Trusts and Workforce Development Confederations have an important role in raising the profile of child protection issues and in enabling opportunities for work-based training.

References

Bannon MJ, Carter YH, Jackson NR, Paice M and Thorne W (2001) Meeting the training needs of GP registrars in child abuse and neglect. *Child Abuse Review* 2001; **10**: 254–61.

Braun D (1993) Training for front-line workers. *Child Abuse Review* **2**: 54–9.

Carter YH (1995) Child Abuse: A Dilemma for General Practice. (Editorial) *Update* January 60–1.

Department of Health (1999) *Working Together to Safeguard Children.* London: HMSO.

Gilardi J (1991) Child protection in a south London district. *Health Visitor* **64**: 225–7.

Hallett C and Birchall E (1992) *Co-ordination and child protection.* London: HMSO.

Hazzard A and Rupp G (1983) Training teachers to identify and intervene with abused children. Cochrane data base.

Hendry E (1997) Engaging general practitioners in child protection training. *Child Abuse Review* **6**: 60–5.

Jayawant S, Rawlinson A, Gibbon F, Price J, Schulte J, Sharples P *et al.* (1998) Subdural haemorrhages in infants: a population based study. *BMJ* **317**: 1558–61.

Johnson CF (1993) Physicians and medical neglect: variables that affect reporting. *Child Abuse and Neglect* **17**: 605–12.

Lawrence LL and Brannen SJ (2000) The impact of physician training on child maltreatment reporting: a multi-specialty study. *Military Medicine* **165**: 607–11.

Lentsch KA and Johnson CF (2000) Do physicians have adequate knowledge of child sexual abuse? The results of two surveys of practising physicians, 1986 and 1996. *Child Maltreatment* **5**: 72–8.

Leventhal J (1999) The challenges of recognizing child abuse: seeing is believing. *JAMA* **281**: 657–9.

Ling M and Luker Karen (2000) A Protecting children: intuition and awareness in the work of health visitors. *Journal of Advanced Nursing* **32**: 572–9.

Offer-Schechter S, Tirosh E and Cohen A (2000) Physical abuse – physicians' knowledge and reporting attitude in Israel. *European Journal of Epidemiology* **16**: 53–8.

Payne D (1999) GPs loath to report abuse. British Medical Journal **318**: 147.

Polnay J and Blair M (1999) Child Protection Training for 6 Ps. A model programme for busy learners. *Child Abuse Review* **8**: 284–8.

Reiniger A, Robinson E and McHugh M (1995) Mandated training of professionals: a means for improving reporting of suspected child abuse. *Child Abuse and Neglect* **19**: 63–9.

Shor R (1998) Pediatricians in Israel: factors which affect the diagnosis and reporting of maltreated children. *Child Abuse and Neglect* **22**: 143–53.

Simpson CM, Simpson RJ, Power KG, Salter A and Williams G (1994) GPs' and health visitors' participation in child protection case conferences. *Child Abuse Review* **3**: 211–30.

Tilden VP, Schmidt TA, Limandri BJ, Chiodo GT, Garland MJ and Loveless PA (1994) Factors that influence clinicians' assessment and management of family violence. *American Journal of Public Health* **84**: 628–33.

Van Haeringen AR, Dadds M and Armstrong KL (1998) The child abuse lottery – will the doctor suspect and report? Physician attitudes towards and reporting of suspected child abuse and neglect. *Child Abuse and Neglect* **22**:159–69.

van Veenendaal E (1993) Child abuse: does disclosing the fact have implications for medical secrecy? *Medicine and Law* **12**: 25–8.

Warner-Rogers JE, Hansen DJ and Spieth LE (1996) The influence of case and professional variables on identification and reporting of physical abuse: a study with medical students. *Child Abuse and Neglect* **20**: 851–66.

Wright RJ, Wright RO, Farnan L and Isaac NE (1999) Response to child abuse in the pediatric emergency department: need for continued education. *Pediatric Emergency Care* **15**: 376–82.

Chapter 6

Physical abuse

Chris Hobbs

Terminology

Physical abuse of children is also referred to as non-accidental injury or battering. The results of physical abuse include injury, permanent physical harm, death and psychological harm.

Spectrum of physical abuse

In many European countries hitting children is outlawed and would be considered abusive. In the UK it remains permissible for parents to hit a child if they use reasonable force. In practice this means that they do not cause an injury e.g. bruises or mark.

How common is physical abuse?

Research has shown that physical methods of controlling children remain popular. In community studies, for example the work of Marjorie Smith from the Institute of Child Health in London, confirmed that 14% of all children suffered severe experiences of physical punishment. Many children including babies suffered regular physical chastisement in the form of hitting (9 out of 10 children are hit at some time), physical restraint or being tied and bound. In the severe group the possibility of permanent physical or psychological harm was present.

Although the usual picture of the disciplinarian father using physical force to discipline the children is ingrained in our thinking, this research revealed that it was the mothers who were responsible for more of this behaviour – even when their greater contact with the children was taken into account.

Risk factors for physical abuse

These involve risks for the family, child, parents and community.
Family:

- Dysfunctional family
- Past history of abuse

- ♦ Family violence – spouse abuse, animal abuse or neglect, elder abuse
- ♦ Marital difficulties.

Child:

- ♦ Boys are physically abused more than girls
- ♦ Unwanted child, born into an unloving or rejecting relationship
- ♦ Child with disability or illness
- ♦ Neglected child
- ♦ Over-investment in child (too high expectations)
- ♦ Difficult behaviour (is this cause or effect?).

Parents:

- ♦ History of abuse as child
- ♦ Poor self image, feel unable to control their children
- ♦ Uninhibited through alcohol or drugs
- ♦ Under stress, acute or chronic
- ♦ Sexual abusers and domestic violence perpetrators
- ♦ Women (usually mothers) abuse more often than men (a range of men may be playing the role of father)
- ♦ Men who are both stronger and more violent inflict the more serious injuries more often.

How common is physical child abuse?

Child Abuse is recognized as a major morbidity for children. The National Commission on the prevention of Child Abuse (1996) broadly defined child abuse:

> Child abuse consists of anything which individuals, institutions, or processes do or fail to do which directly or indirectly harms children or damages their prospects of safe and healthy development into adulthood.

Using this definition, at least 1 million children are harmed each year:

- ♦ At least 150,000 children annually suffer severe physical punishment likely to cause harm to their development.
- ♦ Up to 100,000 children each year have a potentially harmful sexual experience.
- ♦ 350–400,000 children live in an environment which is consistently low in warmth and high in criticism. These children are emotionally neglected and often are also at risk of physical or sexual abuse.
- ♦ 450,000 children are bullied at school at least once per week. Although not traditionally thought of as child abuse, the harm and suffering which peer abuse causes is increasingly recognized.
- ♦ 250,000 children witness violence between parents and carers.

Physical abuse

This includes non-accidental injury of all kinds where the injury is caused as a result of actions or omissions on the part of a carer. Most physical abuse is perpetrated by the carer. Infants and young children are at greatest risk of a severe or fatal outcome.

Fatal outcome most often follows:

- Blunt or shaking injury to the head
- Suffocation (may present as recurrent apnea or sudden infant death)
- Intra-abdominal injury
- Poisoning (e.g. with drugs or salt).

Common injuries in physical abuse

- Bruising (from blows with the hand or use of implements)
- Bites
- Scratches from nails
- Fractures from grabbing or pulling or shaking, blows, kicks, hitting with implements (ribs, metaphyseal, skull or long bone shaft)
- Burns or scald (tap water immersion, thrown or poured liquid, contact from holding against hot object, friction or carpet, cigarette)
- Eye and mouth injuries from blows, burns and other violence.

The approach to diagnosis

Presentation: a direct report/suspicion raised by the child, family, friend, neighbour, childcare professional.

Important points to look for

- Repeated injuries
- Injuries not consistent with the history
- Patterns of injuries
- Signs of neglect including failure to thrive, sexual abuse
- Unusual behaviour by carers.

Features in the history:

1 Injuries not consistent with history;
2 Too many, too severe, wrong kind, distribution and age;
3 Bruising in a young baby, rib fractures, subdural haematoma, multiple fractures;
4 No history of pain e.g. in a scald or fracture;
5 Unreasonable delay e.g. burn or fracture seen several days after 'accident';
6 Denial and defensiveness are common features.

The parents may be aggressive to professional staff who inquires about an injury. This is worrying but may also adversely affect the doctor's ability to assess objectively a situation and take steps to protect the child.

NB delay in seeking help, parental aggression towards staff, and an incidental discovery of an injury are all worrying features of an injury in a child.

How to assess bruising

+ How many bruises are there?

+ Can you obtain consent by parent to look at the whole child?

+ What are the distribution, pattern, sites, sizes and shapes of any bruises?

+ Where are the bruises? (shins, bony prominence, forehead are more likely in accidents).

+ How many bruises does the child have in all? Surveys have found that up to half of all mobile children have at least one bruise and many children had more than one. However more than 10 bruises is unusual and should invite concern.

+ Don't try to age bruises – you are as likely to be wrong as correct. A yellow bruise is 18–24 hours old – not a lot of help in most investigations. Bruises remain for unpredictable lengths of time and can fade at differing rates even when caused contemporaneously and by similar mechanism.

+ What history is offered for these injuries? Is it clear, incident related or vague and general e.g. he falls over a lot, he bruises easily, she's always covered in bruises.

Notes should be detailed with simple drawings showing the site, size and shape of any bruises with a brief comment about any explanation offered for the injury. Most GPs will opt to involve a paediatrician in the assessment of suspected abuse and should know who to contact. A thorough medical examination will include an assessment of the child's growth and development as well as any injury and an examination to check for signs associated with sexual abuse. This usually takes about 45 to 60 minutes per child and is outside the range of services that most GPs choose to offer.

Bruises in abuse

Site: ears, cheeks, eyes, mouth, trunk including chest and abdomen, genitalia, upper or unexposed parts of limbs, softer areas e.g. buttocks, neck should arouse suspicion of ill treatment.

Patterns: two black eyes may result from a hard blow to the forehead (and unless following a road traffic accident is likely to be abusive).

A single black eye requires a penetrating injury to the eye socket and an appropriate history to match. A child who walks into a wall is much more likely to bruise the forehead than to receive a peri-orbital haematoma which may follow a fist in the face.

A hard blow to the face or head with an outstretched hand results in a typical pattern of injury. There is a wrap-around distribution and complex petechial speckling pattern within a broadly parallel linear distribution. The fingers correspond to the unmarked stripes between the rows of petechial haemorrhage.

Grip mark bruises consist of clusters of circular bruises 0.5 to 1.0 cm in diameter around the chest or limbs numbering 2, 3, 4 or 5 per grasp. Try fitting your hand over the bruises. Look for the thumb mark.

Shaken babies may have bruises to the chest wall where grasped and held, but remember as with all injuries where a tight grasp is implied there may or may not be bruises (e.g. limb forced into hot water, a wrenched and fractured limb etc.).

Kick marks may be large, irregular and generally round bruises most often on the legs.

Bites consist of double elliptical crescents of uniform bruising and if fresh, individual teeth marks may be visible. Bite mark identification can assist with perpetrator identification by dental experts. Dog and other animal bites consist of irregular shaped patterns often with areas of broken skin for example where the prominent canines have punctured.

Marks from implements: stick, belt, buckle, shoe and other implements may leave characteristic shapes and patterns. Matching the implement to the injury is the job of the criminal investigation.

Differential diagnosis of bruises:

- Clotting defect e.g. ITP, rarely haemophilia, leukaemia (clotting studies may be required to confirm or exclude);
- Collagen disorder e.g. Ehlers Danlos (rare)
- Congenital lesion e.g. Mongolian blue spot, vascular lesion (common)
- Felt tip pen, paint, clothes dye (this is the commonest – try to wipe off any unusual bruises).

Mouth injuries – many more injuries to the mouth can be detected by careful examination by a trained examiner with dental skills than by a cursory look. The torn frenulum of the upper lip is a good marker for a forceful entry injury. Look for broken teeth and bruises inside the mouth as well.

Fractures

Fractures following child abuse occur most often to infants and toddlers in the age range birth to 2 years.

In the first year of life as many as 4 out of 10 fractures are inflicted or abusive injuries. When infants are immobile the risk of accidental injury decreases so that any injury whether bruise, fracture or burn under the age of around 9 months should attract considerable suspicion.

Although most fractures will reach hospital, many will present initially to doctors in primary care and there may be no history of trauma at presentation.

Keep the possibility of a fracture at the forefront of your mind in a child in the following circumstances:

- Not moving or using limb
- Failure to weight bear
- Pain in limb
- Swelling on head or limb

- Parental concerns re a limb even if clinically normal (fracture healing or healed – late presentation)
- Unusual distress if handled.

Soft boggy swellings on the scalp outside the neonatal period are the result of underlying skull fracture until proved otherwise. This is a useful rule even if there is no history of injury offered.

In infants fractures of the proximal limb bones are strongly linked with abuse – femur and humerus.

Birth injury usually presents at birth or immediately afterwards – the clavicle is the commonest. Beware of other injuries which present later but claimed to be birth injuries. Radiological signs of healing take about 7 to 10 days to appear.

Rib fractures are usually occult but crepitus can occasionally be detected when the chest is gently palpated. Rib fractures along with metaphyseal fractures (fractures through the growing ends of bones) offer strong evidence of abuse. Rib fractures can be difficult to detect on chest x-ray, especially when fresh. Repeated x-ray after 2 weeks improves the number of bony injuries detected in infants. Cardiopulmonary resuscitation in infants does not cause rib fractures.

History with a fracture

Accident: history of sufficient injury (minor fall e.g. from a settee is insufficient to explain a skull or other fracture). Throwing a baby up and catching awkwardly should not cause fracture, minor falling over or downstairs are usually insufficient to cause serious injury.

When a fracture occurs there are pain, distress and immediate recognition of a significant injury. Swelling and loss of function occur rapidly. Presentation to hospital usually follows.

Abuse

The injury is discovered following reports of minor injury or no injury at all. Stories that the child didn't cry are common. 'We put him to bed and he slept all night. The next day his arm was swollen'. Other examples are – 'someone opened a door onto the infant's head', 'he caught his arm being lifted out of the cot/buggy'. Parents may say they noticed a swelling e.g. on the scalp or that the child was not using the affected limb. The child may be presented late when there is little to find clinically as healing may already be advanced and pain and swelling much less. Fractures aged 7 to 10 days or more can be recognized by the presence of subperiosteal new bone formation and callus.

Differential diagnosis of fractures

- Accident
- Abuse
- Birth injury e.g. clavicle, humerus (NB callus at 10 days)

- Neonatal rickets
- Copper deficiency is not now seen in the UK
- Osteogenesis imperfecta: mild Type 1 or 1V – both are rare, a family history is usual and 'blue sclerae' are found in Type 1.
- Although brittle bones are often claimed to be the cause of multiple fractures in an infant, the condition is far less common than physical child abuse. The diagnosis needs to be established on clinical grounds after a careful consideration of all the features.

Burns and scalds

These injuries are viewed as serious abuse, implying in many cases a sadistic element, and can be linked with sexual violence.

Burns are classified according to aetiology:

- Dry, contact usually from hot metal object e.g. fire surround, clothes iron, curling tongs.
- Scald from liquid usually water, steam or food.
- Flame including cigarette from very hot source which burns the tissues and singes hair.
- Friction when a child's body is for example dragged forcefully across a carpeted floor.
- Electrical from the passage of current through the child's skin.
- Microwave – unbelievably there are reports of babies placed in microwave ovens.
- Radiant burns – children forced to stand in front of radiant fires and sunburn – usually neglect.
- Chemical burns from caustic acids and alkalis.

Characteristics of abusive burns

History:

- Unwitnessed incident, vague account, lack of expected responses from child and carer.
- Denial injury is a burn.
- Injury is not consistent with history.
- Repeated burns (such is the distress/misery, that parents usually manage to avoid a second accidental burn injury).

The injury:

- Site: backs of hands, buttocks, soles of feet, face but anywhere. Multiple sites/ multiple contacts e.g. of iron.
- Shape: sharp demarcation lines suggest object held and normal withdrawal reflex impeded.

- Immersion scalds: when the immersion is abusive you may see the forced immersion scald pattern. The features are:
  1 Circumferential uniform scalding around the limb in glove or stocking pattern to depth of immersion.
  2 Tide mark indicates that the limb/buttock was still in the water i.e. forcibly held.
  3 Absent splash marks suggests child did not hurriedly move as expected. Grip mark bruises sometimes seen but not always.
  4 Length of time of immersion can be calculated if temperature of water is known.
  5 Investigation by team including Child Protection Paediatrician, Police, Forensic Science Officer who can take measurements of water temperature, time and depth as per history offered by carer.

Remember bath scalds do not occur in non-impaired adults. Be suspicious of all bath scalds in children. Parents know the dangers of domestic hot water.

Cigarette burns

Deep circular crater, 0.5–1.0 cm. in diameter which scars. Accidental brushed contact results in a superficial injury, roughly circular but with a tail. There is insufficient heat in a hot ash end falling off a cigarette to produce the abusive burn.

Contact burns

Children may be taught not to touch the fire by having their hands held against the hot exterior. Clearly defined grid patterns result. Fireguards are a legal requirement where there are young children living in a house.

Iron burns are common – look for:

- Incredible story (e.g. 2-year-old took iron out of cupboard, plugged it in and burned herself, switched it off and put it away. I noticed it much later.)
- Deep well circumscribed injury e.g. on back of hand
- Parents claim child's hand was trapped by weight of iron which fell on it
- More than one contact
- Unusual site
- Extensive area of contact
- Central heating radiators rarely accidentally burn – temperature is too low and reflex withdrawal protects.

Differential diagnosis of burns:

- Impetigo which may blister, is superficial, has a yellow crust, satellite lesions and does not usually scar
- Nappy rash
- Staphylococcal scalded skin syndrome
- Fungal infection e.g. ring worm can look like a burn.

Head injury

This is the leading cause of death in physical child abuse. The mortality is concentrated in infancy when 4 out of 5 deaths due to trauma are the result of abuse, and 95% of severe head injuries in infancy are due to abuse.

Intracranial damage following accidents is exceptional in falls. Head injury involves either or both shaking and impact injury.

The shaken baby is recognized by a combination of symptoms and signs. About 100 such infants are recognized in the UK each year, so it is not a rare condition.

Many of these children are taken to the GP before the diagnosis is made. The clinical manifestations are variable and there are both acute and chronic presentations.

The main features include:

+ Sudden collapse of previously well infant that becomes apnoeic, may fit looks pale and shocked or may rapidly die;

+ Presence of injury – bruises, swelling to head, fractures of ribs/limbs;

+ Enlarged or enlarging head;

+ Non-specific symptoms of vomiting, gastro-intestinal disturbance, poor feeding, irritability, crying.

Examination may reveal in some, but not all, cases retinal haemorrhages, bruises, full fontanelle, pallor (the Haemoglobin is often low), poor handling.

Radiological investigations confirm the presence of subdural haemorrhage with or without brain swelling/bleeding/other injury. Skeletal survey may reveal skull, limb or rib fractures old or new. The most consistent part of the syndrome is the presence of subdural haemorrhage. The presence of bruising to the scalp, or a fracture of the skull, confirms the presence of a likely impact and although not present in every case has lead to the term 'shaken–impact syndrome'.

The mortality and long term neurological sequelae are considerable. In some cases repeated shaking occurs. This in theory offers the possibility of limiting harm by early detection and intervention. However because of the hidden nature of this problem and the subtle presentation, in many cases diagnosis is delayed in about a third of cases. Doctors should have a high index of suspicion of this condition and include it in the differential diagnosis of any unexplained illness in an infant. The peak age is the first 6 months of life although a similar syndrome has been described in adults who have been shaken.

Urgent admission to hospital is required if this condition is suspected and child protection procedures should be followed. Rare cases of subdural haemorrhage may follow clotting and metabolic disorder, which will need to be excluded.

Other serious injuries include injury to the abdomen from kicks, punches or from standing on the child. Rupture of solid or hollow organs can produce an acute abdomen picture. The lack of a history of trauma and delay in presentation may mean that diagnosis is difficult to make or delayed and mortality consequently high. Although the presence of abdominal bruising is a useful clue it is not present in all cases.

Munchausen syndrome by proxy abuse (MSBP)

This is not a rare or exotic form of child abuse. It is commonly encountered in paediatric practice and the family GP should know all cases.

The syndrome is named after Baron K.F.H. von Munchausen, a German eighteenth-century mercenary whose adventures bore little resemblance to reality. Another term sometimes used but of lesser popularity is factitious illness. The parent who induces, invents, or exaggerates an illness in their child does so for personal gain in the form of sympathy, nurturing, attention, status and respect which they receive from the medical caring team (and society in general which sympathizes with the plight of the parent with an ill child). Publicity and money (e.g. disability allowance) are other gains in some cases.

The first descriptions were based on hospital inpatients, where many of the mothers who perpetrated the abuse had a nursing background and produced elaborate deceptions using medical knowledge. However other cases with less dramatic medical presentations may present, e.g. to primary care teams.

Case history 1

A deprived, poor, single mother took a well child to the casualty department of her local hospital 39 times in a year. When she complained to her GP about her child's feet, he referred her to an orthopaedic surgeon who unnecessarily straightened his toes. She also claimed repeated street assaults on herself for which the police found no basis. At one time she was taking the child to five different paediatric clinics for trivial non-existent conditions. When referred to social services it was found that she had filled her house and garden with cheap broken kitchen appliances leaving little room for herself or the child. The child's behaviour was described as bizarre and other children at school avoided him. The mother was said by a psychiatrist to have a personality disorder.

Case history 2

A single deprived mum complained that her infant fell asleep uncontrollably. GP referred to paediatrician who admitted the child for observation to the ward. Toxicology negative. Major parenting inadequacies. Investigations – including one for melatonin secreting pineal tumour – were extensively undertaken by enthusiastic paediatric staff. Eventually the child was removed to care where symptoms abruptly ceased and the child became entirely normal. On contact with mum, child's behaviour suddenly deteriorated. Care order obtained. It was not clear how the mother induced unconsciousness in her child.

Definition of MSBP abuse

+ Illness fabricated by child's carer
+ Child presented repeatedly for medical care assessment and care

- Perpetrator denies the true aetiology of the child's illness
- Symptoms and signs cease when child is separated form the perpetrator.

Management is always difficult. There will be a number of professionals who sympathize with and may have colluded with the parent's needs and behaviour. This may occur even though the child may appear perfectly well to an experienced doctor.

One junior doctor, after a training course which included this problem, said 'I will never be the same again. I have always believed what parents (and patients) have told me. I now understand that I need to question what I hear and assess situations differently'.

Common Presentations of MSBP abuse

- Poisoning – producing symptoms and illness through the administration of medicines/other poisons
- Suffocation – child presents as sudden unexplained collapse
- Bleeding (haematemesis, malaena, haematuria)
- Fits
- Failure to thrive
- Apnoea
- Diarrhoea and vomiting
- Rashes
- Fever.

Warning signs of MSBP abuse:

- Persistent or recurrent illness (the fat case notes)
- Impossibility of resolving the child's health problems (one goes away, another one appears). Treatment fails to work
- Doctor shopping (includes falling out with doctors)
- Discrepancy between the carer's description and the child's apparent good health
- Overly attentive mother, will not leave child – appears cheerful despite the grave situation
- Several medical opinions – 'collects doctors'.

Why be concerned?

1 Physical consequences of unnecessary investigations and treatments;
2 Emotional problems associated with chronic invalidism, distorted relationships, insecurity and preoccupation with illness;
3 Poor relationships, isolation, lack of normal experiences;
4 Poor education, lack of skills.

The management is more complex than the more usual cases of physical abuse. The primary care team has a crucial role to play as it is often the only agency which has an overview of the extent of health care involvement in these cases. Collecting together what is often extensive information from a number of different sources is a crucial part of the assessment process with which primary health care is involved.

Chapter 7

Neglect and its impact on child welfare

Jocelyn Jones and Anna Gupta

Childhood neglect is a significant and endemic problem in Britain, and it has been underestimated and arguably 'neglected' by child welfare professionals (Minty and Pattinson 1994; Stevenson 1998; Jones and Gupta 1998). In England, registrations for neglect on the Child Protection Register have been increasing steadily, and since 1997 neglect has been the most frequently used category for registration (Department of Health 1999a). Evidence from research shows that neglect can significantly impair children's health and development (Polansky *et al.* 1981; Corby 1993; Minty and Pattinson 1994; Bifulco and Moran 1996), and affect parenting capacity at a later stage (Gaudin 1993; Coohey 1995). This chapter considers the nature of child neglect, and professional responses within the current context of child welfare provision.

Definitions

Child maltreatment is a socially constructed phenomenon and all definitions are open to interpretation and value judgements. Neglect, however, poses particular difficulties. For example, in a study examining different professionals' perceptions of child maltreatment, Birchall and Hallett (1995) found least consensus with respect to definitions of neglect and emotional abuse. The Department of Health (1999b) define neglect in *Working Together to Safeguard Children* as follows:

> Neglect is the persistent failure to meet a child's basic physical and/or psychological needs, likely to result in the serious impairment of the child's health or development. It may involve a parent or carer failing to provide adequate food, shelter and clothing, failing to protect a child from physical harm or danger, or the failure to ensure access to appropriate medical care or treatment. It may also include neglect of, or unresponsiveness to, a child's basic emotional needs.

Although this definition does include specific examples of neglectful behaviours, child welfare professionals need, on a daily basis, to grapple with the application of the terms 'persistent' and 'serious impairment'.

The above definition is associated with the concept of 'significant harm', which is the threshold identified within the Children Act 1989 that justifies compulsory intervention in family life in the best interests of children. The concept of significant harm requires the attribution of the harm to parental care. However, neglect is a complex issue and often the result of a number of interrelated factors, including poverty. Dubowitz *et al.* (1993) propose a definition that focuses on the basic needs of children not being met, and argue that the responsibility for meeting these needs is shared between parents and the wider community. In terms of thresholds for intervention, it is therefore also important for professionals to be aware of Section 17 of the Children Act 1989, which places a duty on local authorities to safeguard and promote the welfare of children in need in their area. Children are deemed to be in need if it is unlikely they would achieve a reasonable standard of health and development without the provision of services.

The definition of neglect contained in *Working Together to Safeguard Children* (Department of Health 1999b) includes emotional neglect. A number of authors have identified the links between neglect and other forms of child maltreatment. Dent (1996) states that neglect can comprise emotional and physical elements, and utilizes attachment theory to suggest that 'an emotionally neglecting parent can perform acts of both omission and commission because of a lack of benevolence towards the child'.

Child Protection: Messages from Research (Department of Health 1995) identifies families that are low on warmth and high on criticism as being potentially harmful for children. It is suggested that chronicity and severity are important factors in determining the level of harm experienced by the children. In families that are low on warmth and high on criticism 'negative incidents accumulate as if to remind a child that he or she is unloved' and the risk of physical neglect, physical and, occasionally sexual abuse is probably at its highest (Department of Health 1995).

The effects of neglect

There are considerable methodological problems associated with research on the effects of child neglect. In particular, it is difficult to differentiate between factors that are consequences of neglect and those associated with poverty and deprivation (Parton 1995). However there is general agreement that neglect has a detrimental effect on the development of children. Gaudin (1993), in his review of the research on this subject, concluded that 'child neglect can have devastating effects on the intellectual, physical, social and psychological development of children'.

Much of the research considers the effect of physical abuse and neglect, highlighting adverse effects on emotional development including low self-esteem and problems forming attachments. Difficulties in social and intellectual functioning, such as in forming peer relationships and school performance, have also been identified. In the longer term, links have been suggested between abuse and neglect in childhood and maternal depression, drug abuse, offending behaviour and general adjustment to life (Corby 1993; Bifulco and Moran 1998).

Studies have shown that deficiencies in development seem to be more common in children who were neglected rather than those who were physically abused only (Minty and Pattinson 1994). Dent (1996) suggests that the available evidence demonstrates that children who experience neglect 'have the most serious school related difficulties and that the signs of cognitive and socio-emotional delays manifest themselves at a very young age'. A study that evaluated the quality of parenting in families where there was physical abuse, found a predominant style that was characterized not by aggression nor over-control, but rather by inconsistency, laxity and unresponsiveness (Pitcairn *et al.* 1993). Many of these children were assessed as being highly disturbed, which tended to support research which suggests that such styles of parenting lead to aggressive and behavioural difficulties in the children. Egeland and colleagues (1983) found that the neglected children:

> Appeared to have difficulty in pulling themselves together to deal with tasks . . . They were the least flexible and creative in attempts to solve (a particular) task. Children in the neglect without physical abuse group received the lowest ratings in both self-esteem and agency (i.e. appropriate confidence and assertiveness). These children were also the most dependent and demonstrated the lowest ego control in their pre-school.
>
> (Egeland *et al.* 1983 p. 469)

The inquiry report into the death of Paul (Bridge Child Care Consultancy Service 1995) provides a summary of some of the effects of neglect. It states that:

> Babies and children who are physically and emotionally neglected are at high risk of suffering:
>
> - Gross under-stimulation
> - Failure to thrive, which can lead to poor growth, developmental delay and in an extreme form, death
> - Disturbances in emotional attachment
> - Language delay
> - Conduct disorder
> - Poor educational performance
> - Severe nappy rash and other skin infections
> - Recurrent and persistent minor infections.
>
>   As they grow older they will feel:
>
> - Unloved and unloving
> - Powerless and hopeless
> - A severe lack of self-esteem
> - Isolated from their peers.

This list of the consequences of child neglect is a timely reminder of the importance of early identification and intervention in this field, thus putting an end to 'professional neglect' of neglect.

Factors associated with child neglect

It is now widely recognized that child abuse is a multifactorial phenomenon, involving a dynamic interplay of individual, familial and societal factors. The literature highlights a wide range of factors associated with neglect. A major factor associated with neglect is poverty. Most cases of neglect that come to the attention of child welfare agencies are from the most deprived sections of our society. It is often difficult to separate early indicators of neglect from those of widespread social disadvantage and poverty (Parton 1995). A recent major study on poverty and social exclusion in Britain (Gordon *et al.* 2000) highlights the desperate plight of many poor families in Britain today. Some of the findings include:

- Roughly 17% of households cannot afford adequate housing conditions as perceived by the majority of the population, i.e. they cannot afford to keep their home adequately heated, free from damp or in a decent state of decoration.

- About 33% of British children go without at least one of the things they need, like three meals a day, toys, out of school activities or adequate clothing. 18% of children go without two or more items or activities defined as necessities by the majority of the population.

Although the majority of families living in poverty do not neglect their children, the unrelenting stress of social deprivation and exclusion can in some families manifest itself in the neglect of children's basic needs (NCH Action for Children 1996; Stevenson 1998).

Childhood adversity in parents' backgrounds is also associated with neglect. The Bridge report into the death of Paul (1996) asserts that:

> The children at greatest risk are those where the adult's own childhood was abusive or neglectful, resulting either in an inability to recognise the needs of their own children or the development of a need to impose their will at the expense of their own children.

This can then have an impact on the support offered to parents by their wider family. Gaudin (1993) suggests that the social networks of neglectful mothers tend to be dominated by relatives who are critical rather than supportive. Coohey (1995) concludes that 'mothers of neglectful mothers when compared with others, are either less willing or less able to give emotional support to their neglectful daughters and neglectful daughters are less interested in receiving emotional support'.

Two studies have considered the factors associated with families that have come within the remit of child protection practice in Britain. Stone's study in 1998 confirmed that neglect was multifactorial. After considering factors relating to parents/ caregivers, he concluded that a large proportion were significantly damaged and disadvantaged people, who were ill-equipped emotionally and practically, to care for children. The study confirmed the importance of emotional/relationship factors as well as poverty and deprivation.

Similarly Allsop and Stevenson (1995) highlight characteristics of cases where there were components of neglect and which the social workers in their study found particularly complex and challenging. These families were mostly living in poverty; mostly single parents; nearly all had a long relationship with social services and in the majority the parenting was hovering on the edge of 'not good enough'.

Certain parental behaviour, such as substance misuse, is seen as a major contributing factor of child neglect (Swadi 1994). Cleaver and colleagues (1999) reviewed the literature on the impact of parental mental illness, problem alcohol and drug use, and domestic violence on children's development. They concluded that there are many ways these problems can impact adversely on parents' abilities to meet their children's needs which include the neglect of physical needs, attachment problems and increased risk of separation. Forrester (2000) also found a strong relationship between parental substance misuse and child protection registration for neglect.

Turney (2000) highlights the gendered nature of the discussion about neglect. She suggests that as ideas about care and nurture are strongly linked with the feminine in Western culture, neglect tends to be viewed as an absence of female care, i.e. something that specifically *mothers* do (or don't do). Tanner and Turney (2000) express concern that a response based on stereotypical assumptions about women's roles and capacities will fail to recognize the complex realities of neglect. They argue that neglect stems from a breakdown in the child's main caring relationship. Professionals must be aware of the range of stressors, (e.g. poverty, domestic violence, racism and depression), that can impact on a mother's ability to care and take account of the range of relationships that are significant in families where neglect is a key feature.

There is currently no evidence to suggest that serious neglect is more common in any one ethnic group. However, there are clearly differences in values and norms in child-rearing practices between cultures (Korbin 1991). Stevenson (1998) explains that there is a serious dearth of literature that explores the definition and application of the concept of neglect to diverse ethnic and cultural groups in Britain. She cautions that workers when making judgements about what is 'good enough' standards of care should not fall into either extreme of *cultural dogmatism* ('ours is the best way') or *cultural relativism* ('anything goes').

Decision-making in cases of child neglect

The inherent nature of child neglect poses particular difficulties for professionals making decisions about how to help families. For much of the last twenty years in Britain there has been an increase in poverty and deprivation, but a corresponding decrease in the resources of child welfare agencies (Parton 1995). Families referred for neglect are often living in circumstances characterized by poverty and deprivation. The report into the death of Paul draws on the work of Rosenberg and Cantwell (1993). They argue that a distinction must be made between neglect caused by material poverty, which can be alleviated by financial help, and that caused by emotional poverty. These may both exist within families, but relief of the material poverty does not relieve emotional poverty. In the current climate of limited resources such distinctions are not easily made, and the difficulties facing practitioners deciding when and how to intervene in cases of child neglect are compounded.

The balance that practitioners need to achieve is to support and empower parents whilst still maintaining the child's welfare as being paramount. Workers can, through their identification with the oppressed position of the parent, lose sight of the needs of the child. Given the multiple problems many neglectful parents face, their needs can frequently dominate and they become the primary client. In a system where issues of blame and guilt are central, workers can find it hard to make judgements about the culpability of vulnerable and disadvantaged parents (Stevenson 1996). In addition the chronic nature of neglect and professional 'acclimatization' to poor standards of care over time, make it difficult to decide when a situation has reached a 'point of no return' and compulsory intervention is necessary. The wider context of child welfare provision may further compound difficulties of decision-making in cases of neglect (Jones and Gupta 1998).

The social, political and organizational context

During the later half of the 1970s, 1980s and early 1990s, child protection professionals were primarily focused on identifying physical abuse. Following the Cleveland Inquiry (Butler-Sloss 1988), their attention was directed towards child sexual abuse. Hence the plight of children experiencing childhood neglect was ignored by practitioners, policy makers and academics (Minty and Pattinson, 1994; Stevenson, 1996). A number of factors contributed to this oversight:

◆ Public inquiries into child abuse and subsequent scapegoating of social workers;

◆ Policy decisions of the Conservative government which led to substantial reductions in resources to public services;

◆ An increasing role for the police in the management of the child protection system (Jones and Gupta 1998).

Within this context, it was the risk management model of child protection procedures that predominated. Risk is defined as danger from a well-specified, adverse outcome, with the focus on safety rather than welfare (Allsop and Stevenson 1995).

In 1995, the Department of Health published *Child Protection: Messages from Research*, a document that summarized the key findings from 20 research studies into the child protection system. A number of important themes emerged about the child protection process. These included an overemphasis on investigations of incidents of abuse without considering the wider needs and context of the child's life. While vulnerable children and families were referred to the child protection system, many did not receive support, as they did not fulfil the threshold for child protection registration. One study conducted by Gibbons *et al.* (1995) found that 17%–32% of referrals to the statutory authorities resulted from neglect. In comparison with physical and sexual abuse, referrals for neglect were much less likely to reach the conference stage. Of the 66 substantiated referrals identified as being in the highest risk category, 36 (54%) were not conferenced. Aldgate and Tunstill (1995), confirmed that children who were referred to the child protection agencies as being 'in need' as opposed to having been abused received little or no service.

A study that considered 43 cases identified as being of concern because of physical abuse, found that the parenting styles of many of the respondents could be characterized as being neglectful. However, the focus of intervention was on prevention of further injuries, rather than on the harm caused by the day-to-day parenting of their carers (Pitcairn *et al.* 1993). The studies by Minty and Pattinson (1994) and Allsop and Stevenson (1995) found that even when cases of neglect were identified, social workers had particular difficulties making decisions about when a situation had reached the 'point of no return' and compulsory intervention was necessary.

Messages from Research (Department of Health 1995), triggered a widespread debate about the nature of child welfare provision, often referred to as the 'refocusing initiative'. The need to increase family support services to children in need was recognised, as was the importance of viewing children involved in the child protection process as 'children in need where there may be a protection problem'. The publication of the *Framework for the Assessment of Children in Need and their Families* (Department of Health 2000) was a significant development in the changing context of child welfare provision, as it offered opportunities for improving service delivery to children experiencing neglect. However, it is important to acknowledge that many problems arise from insufficient resources and staff shortages. In addition poverty and deprivation remain a key feature of many children's lives in Britain in the beginning of the twenty-first century (Gordon *et al.* 2000).

Assessment and intervention

The Framework for the Assessment of Children in Need and their Families (Department of Health 2000) outlines a mechanism whereby all professionals working with children and families may determine whether a child is in need under the Children Act 1989 and decide how best to help. The framework is a particularly useful tool for assessing neglect, as it requires an assessment of a child's developmental needs, parenting capacity, and wider family and environmental factors. It is based on the ecological approach that suggests that 'an understanding of a child must be located within the context of the child's family (parents or caregivers and the wider family) and of the community and culture in which he or she is growing up' (Department of Health 2000). Other writers have also suggested that an ecological model is a useful model for undertaking a systematic assessment of the complex interactions between family members, the local community and wider society when considering neglect, particularly as issues such as poverty, racism and social isolation often characterize the lives of many families (Stevenson 1998; Tanner and Turney 2000).

The widened scope of service provision to include all children in need offers the possibility that increased levels of support will be offered to families where children may be experiencing neglect not necessarily attributable to parental harm, and those where preventative services may reduce the need for more coercive interventions (Thoburn *et al.* 2000). In this respect policy initiatives in Britain are becoming more similar to those in other countries of Europe, where child protection and child welfare work are synonymous (Cooper *et al.* 1995).

A detailed analysis of the information gathered during an assessment is crucial. The guidance on the Assessment Framework stresses the importance of practitioners utilizing relevant theory and research to underpin their decisions (Department of Health 2000). Stevenson (1998 p. 63) provides some guidance:

> Seek to understand the meaning of the problematic or unacceptable behaviour to the adult concerned; *for example*: a very dirty house. Meaning: a depressed mother? A mother in poor physical health? A mother overwhelmed by too many young children? A mother who feels dirty and debased herself? All of these? Some of these? *For example*: a mother's seeming insensitivity towards a baby crying. Meaning: no experience of being nurtured?

Therefore, not understanding that she is needed? Depressed, unable to respond at that time? Uncertainty as to what is needed? Anger towards the child? (Why?)

An assessment that explores the complex and dynamic interplay of individual, familial and societal factors which frame the lives of many neglectful families is likely to lead to a multifaceted plan of intervention by a number of professionals. These may include practical support, parenting skills training, family and individual therapeutic work, nursery provision respite care, and the strengthening of informal support networks (Gaudin 1993; Stevenson 1998). Stevenson (1998) also expresses a cautionary note when she states that it is difficult to effect change in seriously neglectful carers, and for some children substitute care will be essential to safeguard and promote their welfare.

Inter-agency work

An inter-agency approach to assessment and provision of services is essential in cases of child neglect and is required by government guidance (Department of Health 1999, 2000a). Health visitors occupy a key position in being able to identify young children experiencing neglect and provide early intervention. They should be able to share vital information on the child's developmental needs and parenting capacity in the assessment process. Health visitors also have a pivotal role in the provision of ongoing support and monitoring of young children. Similarly, the family's general practitioner should be involved in the identification and intervention with neglectful families, especially as many parents may be experiencing mental health and substance misuse problems. Teachers are in regular contact with children and are therefore well placed to identify cases of child neglect. Thoburn *et al.* (2000) found that apart from 'inadequate supervision', referrals for emotional abuse and neglect were evenly distributed between health professionals, schools and the families themselves. The police most frequently made referrals for 'inadequate supervision'. Other professionals, not least adult mental health and substance misuse workers, also play important roles with families where children may be experiencing neglect.

Although Britain has a highly developed system for interagency and interprofessional cooperation, research reveals many tensions and difficulties, most of which are relevant to cases of neglect. There are clearly aspects of the political and social context that work against effective communication and cooperation, such as frequent organizational change and fragmentation. In addition the complex nature of child neglect appears to exacerbate some of the problems likely to be present due to professionals' different value and knowledge bases, roles and organizational systems. Birchall with Hallett's (1995) detailed study found that:

Physical and sexual abuse are evidently rated more severely than the other categories by all the professions. Within (all) the categories, it is clearly more difficult to establish either internal or interprofessional consensus about cases less severe. This must cause problems in establishing a baseline for protective intervention. As was expected, cases of neglect and emotional abuse cause most dissensus. Of cases generally, there is total interprofessional consensus in only a minority of cases but there are many areas of agreement within and between the professionals which should support a considerable degree of consensual action.

All child welfare agencies need to constantly improve working relationships with other professionals. Joint training that seeks to develop a common definition and understanding of neglect as well as the development of common protocols and policies represent important initiatives.

Conclusion

Chronic and severe childhood neglect cause significant harm to children. The impairment of children's health and development is likely to effect self-esteem and resilience to cope with adversity; this in turn may impact on the ability to function effectively as adults and parents. However, as Gaudin (1993) points out, whilst several studies do point to a cycle of neglect, the direct cause–effect relationship between parental history of neglect and subsequent neglect of children is not clearly established. There are several 'important mediating factors' for victims of neglect who do not repeat the cycle, such as 'fewer stressful life events, stronger more stable and supportive relationships with husbands and boyfriends; physically healthier babies'. They are also less likely to be maltreated by both parents and more apt to have reported a supportive relationship with one parent or with another adult. These mediating factors provide critical indicators for improving parents' potential.

The message from this research is that professionals must consider parenting capacity within both an historical and community context, addressing both negative and positive factors in the past and present. Thus, a window of albeit modest opportunity to effect change, building on potential mediating factors, is enabled. The medical model of prevention at primary, secondary and tertiary levels is useful in identifying different types of activity aimed at prevention of child neglect. Gough (1993) outlines the three levels as:

◆ Primary: interventions aimed at 'whole' populations

◆ Secondary: interventions aimed at individuals or groups considered to be at risk

◆ Tertiary: reactive interventions concerned to prevent unwanted events recurring.

Stevenson (1998) urges some caution in adapting such a model to the social welfare field, although Hardiker *et al.* (1991a, 1991b) and Hardiker (1999) have most usefully developed such a framework to describe levels of intervention in child welfare.

Childcare professionals are in an ideal position to identify children and families in need of *second level* intervention. These include families in temporary crisis or early difficulties. The aim is to restore personal and social functioning so that direct interventions by social services are no longer required. In their study on family support in cases of emotional maltreatment and neglect, Thoburn and colleagues (2000) highlight the need for professionals to provide services at an early stage of problem formation as many families are highly likely to succumb to stresses at a later stage, by which time the children would be more significantly harmed and harder to help. It also needs to be recognized that for some families whose problems are so entrenched and complex, a long-term package of support will be required and in a minority, the children's welfare will not be able to be safeguarded in their family home and placement in substitute care will be necessary (third level).

Finally, we have to remind ourselves of the holistic nature of human needs, whether as babies, children, young people or adults in their role as parents. As professionals employed in the field of child welfare, we need to strive for opportunities to develop and support multiservice interventions where professionals work in close cooperation within the community, offering an holistic and local service to children and parents. Such a child-focused and inter-professional approach, constructed around the Assessment Framework (Department of Health 2000), is the way forward for all those who are committed to the prevention of child neglect in the twenty-first century.

References

Aldgate J and Tunstill J (1995) *Making Sense of Section 17*. London: HMSO.

Allsop M and Stevenson O (1995) *Social Workers' Perceptions of Risk in Child Protection (A discussion paper)*. University of Nottingham: School of Social Studies.

Bifulco A and Moran P (1998) *Wednesday's Child: Research into Women's Experience of Neglect and Abuse in Childhood and Adult Depression*. London: Routledge.

Birchall E and Hallett C (1995) *Working Together in Child Protection*. London: HMSO.

Bridge Child Care Consultancy Service (1995) *Paul: Death through Neglect*. LONDON: Islington Area Child Protection Committee.

Butler-Sloss E (1988) *Report of the Inquiry into Child Abuse in Cleveland*. London: HMSO.

Cleaver H, Unell I and Aldgate J (1999) *Children's Needs – Parenting Capacity: The Impact of Parental Mental Illness, Problem Alcohol and Drug Use, and Domestic Violence on Children's Development*. London: The Stationery Office.

Coohey C (1995) Neglectful mothers, their mothers and partners: the significance of mutual aid. *Child Abuse and Neglect* 19(8): 885–95.

Cooper A, Hetherington R, Baistow K, Pitts J and Spriggs A (1995) *Positive Child Protection: A view from Abroad*. Dorset: Russell House Publishing.

Corby B (1993) *Child Abuse: Toward a Knowledge Base*. Bukcingham: Open University Press.

Dent RJ (1996) Neglect: its effect on children and young people – an educational perspective, in M Pritchard (ed.) *Neglect: A Fifty Year Search for Answers*. London: The Bridge Child Care Development Service and Islington Area Child Protection Committee.

Department of Health (1995) *Child Protection: Messages From Research*. London: HMSO.

Department of Health (1999a) *Children and Young People on Child Protection Registers*. London: Government Statistical Service.

Department of Health (1999b) *Working Together to Safeguard Children*. London: The Stationery Office.

Department of Health (2000) *Framework for the Assessment of Children in Need and their Families*. London: The Stationery Office.

Dubowitz H, Black M, Starr RH and Zuravin S (1993) A conceptual definition of child neglect. *Criminal Justice and Behaviour* 20(1): 8–26.

Egeland B, Stroufe A and Erikson M (1983) The developmental consequences of different patterns of maltreatment. *Child Abuse and Neglect* 7: 459–69.

Forrester D (2000) Parental substance misuse and child protection in a British sample. *Child Abuse Review* 9: 235–46.

Gaudin J (1993) *Child Neglect: A Guide for Intervention*. National Centre on Child Abuse and Neglect (US Department of Health and Human Services).

Gibbons J, Conroy S and Bell C (1995) *Operating the Child Protection System*. London: HMSO.

Gordon D *et al*. (2000) *Poverty and Social Exclusion in Britain*. York: Joseph Rowntree Foundation.

Gough DA (1993) *Child Abuse Interventions: A Review of Research literature*. London: HMSO.

Hardiker P (1999) Children still in need, indeed: prevention across five decades, in O. Stevenson (ed) *Child Welfare in the UK: Working Together for Young People and their Families*. Oxford: Blackwell Science.

Hardiker P, Exton K and Barker M (1991a) *Policies and Practices in Preventive Child Care*. Aldershot: Avebury.

Hardiker P, Exton K and Barker M (1991b) The social policy contexts of prevention in child care. *British Journal of Social Work* 21: 341–60.

Jones J and Gupta A (1998) The context of decision-making in cases of child neglect. *Child Abuse Review* 7(2): 97–110.

Korbin J (1991) Cross cultural perspectives and research directions for the twenty-first century. *Child Abuse and Neglect* 15(Suppl. 1): 67–77.

Minty B and Pattinson G (1994) The nature of child neglect. *British Journal of Social Work* 24: 733–47.

NCH Action for Children (1996) Children still in need: refocusing child protection in the context of children in need. NCH Action for Children.

Parton N (1995) Neglect as child protection: the political context and practical outcomes. *Children and Society* 9(1): 67–89.

Pitcairn T, Waterhouse L, McGhee J, Secker J and Sullivan C (1993) Evaluating parenting in physical abuse, in L. Waterhouse *Child Abuse and Child Abusers: Prevention and Protection*. London: Jessica Kingsley.

Polansky N, Chalmers M, Williams DP and Werthan Buttenweiser E (1981) *Damaged Parents: An Anatomy of Child Neglect*. Chicago: University of Chicago Press.

Rosenberg D and Cantwell H (1993) The consequences of neglect – individual and societal, in CJ Hobbs, JM Wynne (eds) *Child Abuse*. London: Bailliere Tindall.

Stevenson O (1996) Emotional abuse and neglect: a time for reappraisal. *Child and Family Social Work* 1:13–18.

Stevenson O (1998) *Neglected Children: Issues and Dilemmas*. Oxford: Blackwell Science.

Stone B (1998) Child neglect: practitioners perspectives. *Child Abuse Review* 7: 87–96.

Swadi H (1994) Parenting capacity and substance misuse: an assessment scheme. *Association of Child Psychology and Psychiatry Review and Newsletter* 16(5): 237–44.

Tanner K and Turney D (2000) Observation in the assessment of child neglect. *Child Abuse Review* 9: 337–48.

Thoburn J, Wilding J and Watson J (2000) *Family Support in cases of Emotional Maltreatment and Neglect*. London: The Stationery Office.

Turney D (2000) The feminising of neglect. *Child and Family Social Work* 5: 47–56.

Chapter 8

Emotional abuse

Alyson Hall

Emotional abuse is probably the most difficult form of child abuse for any professional to recognize because there are no obvious physical signs and the child does not usually say anything to any one which might draw attention to his difficulties. The abnormal aspects of parenting or caring which may cause significant harm to children are seen to a lesser extent in many, if not most families, at different points in time. The line between worrying behaviour on the part of parents and emotional abuse is ill-defined and, except in extreme cases, a decision to intervene can usually only be made after concerns persist.

It has long been recognized that emotional abuse is commonly found in conjunction with most forms of child abuse, but it is relatively infrequently recorded on the child protection register as the sole category, especially at the time of initial referral. Nevertheless the most serious and enduring effects of abuse on the child's development and behaviour are now considered to be the result of psychological maltreatment or emotional neglect rather than physical abuse and neglect (Skuse and Bentovim 1994).

Even when it is clear that a parent's behaviour toward a child is emotionally abusive, it is generally more difficult than with other types of abuse for the individual professional to decide if, when, and how to intervene. The decision to initiate child protection procedures is usually taken when several professionals have observed abusive interactions and their effects on the child over a period of time. In practice however child protection procedures for emotional abuse may be initiated following an incident of physical or sexual abuse if, while investigating this or subsequently working with the family, it emerges that emotional abuse remains the principle concern.

Emotional abuse most commonly occurs as a result of repeated patterns of relationships sufficiently abnormal to produce enduring effects on the child's behaviour and emotional development (Thompson and Kaplan 1996). A single or infrequent event, however distressing, is unlikely to produce longstanding harmful effects if the child has secure loving and consistent relationships with his parents. Indeed in well functioning families children are more likely to show distress when a parent acts uncharacteristically harshly or temporarily ignores the child. In contrast, a child who has grown up with sufficiently adverse parenting to show abnormal development or seriously disturbed behaviour may remain very loyal to the parent and show no overt distress. Emotional abuse is therefore most easily recognized by those who are likely to observe a parent's relationship with their child over a long period or at regular intervals. Alternatively of course the child's behaviour may become so abnormal that this leads to professional intervention.

Definition

Although in recent years there has been extensive research in the field of sexual abuse and neglect, as well as physical abuse, there is still very little in the literature about emotional abuse. In the United States of America emotional abuse is still not officially recognized in all States as a form of abuse, but it has been a formal category for registration on the child protection register in the United Kingdom since 1980 (Fogarty 1980).

The original definition used in *Protecting Children* published before the Children Act, was useful in its simplicity:

> The severe adverse effect on the behaviour and emotional development of a child caused by persistent or severe emotional ill-treatment or rejection.

These guidelines acknowledged that all abuse involves some emotional ill-treatment but recommended that children should only be placed on the child protection register for emotional abuse when it was the main or sole form of abuse. At that time a category for registration called 'grave concern' was also available, the use of which was often more straightforward for children who were emotionally abused or neglected.

In contrast, in 1991 a whole edition of the journal *Developmental Psychopathology* (Cicchetti 1991) was devoted to a debate about the definition of psychological maltreatment. This did not succeed in providing much more clarity for practitioners, but it did highlight the growing interest in the problem, the difficulties with definition and intervention and the need for more research. In recent years, partly driven by the political and economic cost to society, the effects of adverse parenting, domestic conflict and the development of conduct disorder in children, together with the evaluation of interventions, have become the focus of research on both sides of the Atlantic.

The current generally accepted definition is that included in the latest child protection guidance, Working Together to Safeguard Children (Department of Health 1999), for use by all agencies involved with children:

> Emotional abuse is the persistent emotional ill-treatment of a child such as to cause severe and persistent adverse effects on the child's emotional development. It may involve conveying to children that they are worthless or unloved, inadequate, or valued only insofar as they meet the needs of another person. It may feature age or developmentally inappropriate expectations being imposed on children. It may involve causing children to feel frightened or in danger, or the exploitation or corruption of children. Some level of emotional abuse is involved in all types of ill-treatment of a child, though it may occur alone.

In England and Wales in 2000, 18% of children were registered for emotional abuse as the sole category. In one deprived inner city borough the percentage of children registered for emotional abuse as a sole category has remained between 12–14% since 1990, although the number of registrations for more than one form of abuse has been steadily increasing. Neglect alone has remained the most frequent category at one third to half of cases but, during 2000, 12% of registrations were for emotional abuse with physical abuse and 12% for emotional abuse combined with neglect. Cases of both neglect and emotional abuse remain on the child protection register for longer periods. This means that these categories are over-represented compared with initial registrations.

Nature of disturbed relationships

There are many forms of parent–child interaction which, if persistent, are characteristically harmful to children. Some will be more apparent than others to the health visitor or general practitioner who has intermittent contact with the family. There are parents who are quite adept at saying and doing what they know is expected of them for relatively short periods in the health centre or during a short home visit, especially once child protection concerns have been raised.

Emotional abuse includes acts of commission, conscious and deliberate in extreme cases, but more often involves unconscious patterns of behaviour which repeat the adults' own experiences in childhood. It also includes acts of omission such as lack of emotional stimulation or responsiveness. There is a lack of clarity in child protection procedures as to whether such emotional neglect should be categorized as neglect or emotional abuse. In practice, when associated with physical neglect it will usually be recorded as neglect, but when associated with other features of emotional abuse it should be recorded as such. By the time sufficient concerns have been identified for child protection procedures to be initiated for either emotional abuse or neglect, the professionals will often have observed several types of harmful interaction. These may justifiably fall into two or more child protection categories and may be recorded as such if persistent or severe enough.

Seven typical patterns of harmful behaviour were proposed by Gabarino et al. (1986) and Hart and Brassard (1987). A category of *developmentally inappropriate interaction* has subsequently been added (Glaser 1993), but these categories have generally been accepted following discussion and some elaboration. They are listed below, together with the frequencies found in a British study of adults who reported that they had been emotionally abused as children (Doyle 1997).

1 *Fear inducing, terrorising or inducing insecurity 95%* – threatening to hurt, kill, or abandon, leaving a child unattended or repeatedly with strangers;

2 *Developmentally inappropriate roles 92%* – using the child to care for the parent, age-inappropriate exposure, excessive responsibilities, overprotection, infantilization;

3 *Rejecting 86%* – scapegoating, actively refusing to respond to the child, making the child feel unloved or worthless;

4 *Isolating 54%* – confining a child to a room alone, locking out of the home, refusing contact with peers;

5 *Degrading 53% or tormenting 18%* – public humiliation, verbal abuse, vindictive teasing;

6 *Ignoring 28%* – caregiver detached, uninvolved, fails to respond sensitively to the child's emotional and developmental needs;

7 *Corrupting or mis-socializing 19%* – encouraging the involvement in drug misuse, criminality, sexual activity, verbal or physical abuse;

8 *Exploiting 0%* – child used for adult's advantage or for profit e.g. pornography, prostitution.

Another British study of 94 children placed on the child protection register for emotional abuse (Glaser and Prior 1997) reported that 42% had been involved in developmentally inappropriate interactions, 34% had experienced rejection or denigration, 27% emotional deprivation and 27% repeated separations. Terrorizing, corrupting or using the child for the emotional needs of the parent were relatively rare. The difference between what professionals are able to identify occurring to abused children and what abused adults retrospectively report of their experiences in childhood is striking, and highlights the difficulties involved in investigating emotional abuse.

Common contexts for emotional abuse

Inconsistency

This is one of the most common problems of parenting, present to varying degrees in all families, but was not included in the original attempts to classify types of emotional abuse (McGee and Wolfe 1991). What parent is never inconsistent? Indeed lack of inconsistency would imply a degree of rigidity and insensitivity that in itself would also be emotionally abusive. It is becoming increasingly clear however that extremes of inconsistency produce serious effects, particularly in the production of aggressive behaviour in children (Patterson *et al.* 1989).

The most common type of inconsistent parenting involves the failure to set appropriate limits. The parent is unable to control the child, giving attention when he is misbehaving, rewarding tantrums by giving him what he wants and, at the same time, ignoring good behaviour. The child may also become adept at playing one parent off against the other. In time the child may come to be perceived by the parent as innately bad and not susceptible to change. This lets the parent off the hook and justifies their increasing anger or rejection of the child. To add to the confusion the parent may be the first to attack a teacher or onlooker for intervening when the child misbehaves. The most difficult and harmful scenario occurs when the child becomes wildly out of control at home and at school, yet the parent fails to see either the behaviour or their own management of it as representing a problem.

Inconsistency of emotional responsiveness

The effect of inconsistent behavioural management is particularly damaging when coupled with pervasive inconsistency of emotional responsiveness. Amongst the group of very disturbed children who are taken into care primarily as a result of emotional abuse, parenting is often characterized by expressions of affection or material indulgence one minute followed by anger, hostility or rejection the next.

Exposure to domestic violence or conflict

Another common form of adverse parenting especially harmful to children, is exposure to domestic violence or conflict between adults in the home. This produces insecurity, distress and, in boys especially, severe behaviour problems (Pynoos and Eth 1986; Rushton 2000). The son of a violent father may become particularly identified with his father from an early age and considered by his mother to be beyond redemption. Conflict may continue long after parental separation, sometimes exacerbated and prolonged by the adversarial legal system. Emotional abuse is present when parents continue to expose and involve their children in their own conflict to such an extent that their emotional development is adversely affected.

It is surprising how long extreme domestic violence can be concealed from social services and from primary care staff who are already involved with the family. The police may be called or neighbours report their concerns but many women refuse to press charges. They often conceal the cause of their injuries. Subsequently, after separation from an abusive partner, they reveal that they were afraid to tell anyone because of the risk of further abuse, fear of losing their children or sheer humiliation. Similarly, children may also be too afraid to disclose what is going on until they have been removed from the situation or the violent partner has left. The mother may not appreciate that exposure to serious conflict, with or without violence, is in itself harmful when the abusive partner does not physically harm the children. They may continue in a violent relationship because their partner is 'a good father' as well as because of their own dependency needs. They have generally experienced abuse themselves in childhood and find it hard to distinguish between the physical and emotional effects of abuse.

In addition, there is another form of emotional abuse that is on a continuum with factitious illness or Munchausen's syndrome by proxy at one extreme and, at the other, excessive anxiety about a child's health. This phenomenon poses significant problems for health professionals, in particular the general practitioner. The child's mother appears to meet her own needs by seeking medical consultations, investigations and treatment for a variety of conditions with respect to the child that may or may not exist. This includes common conditions, the diagnosis of which mainly depends on the parent's history, such as epilepsy, constipation and asthma. If the child is given unnecessary treatment, repeated investigations or is kept away from school, then this constitutes emotional abuse. Even when the underlying problem between the parent and child is recognized, this form of abuse is extremely difficult to manage. Admission to hospital may be helpful in order to observe the child's symptoms and the parent's behaviour.

Characteristics of parents who may be emotionally abusive

Characteristic attitudes and beliefs are frequently observed in abusive parents that underpin their difficulties in parenting. They tend to perceive their children and their behaviour more negatively over time than other parents do. They may consider one child as innately bad or, for example, rigidly see their children as stubborn or irritable and are unwilling to understand their behaviour as a response to other factors such as tiredness or a need for attention. They find it hard to recognize positive behaviour and even harder to hold on to positive attributes over time. They generally remain negative and critical even when the child responds to improved management on their part or to treatment (Trowell *et al.* 1997). Thus they feel they have very little power over their children and see their children as exerting power over them. Common behaviours such as crying are perceived negatively and taken personally. Even a young baby may be experienced as deliberately 'winding them up'. Abusive parents appear to respond unusually aversively to cries of a certain pitch (Crowe and Zeskind 1992).

As already indicated, most forms of emotionally abusive behaviour occur on a continuum with less severe but common negative interactions between parents and their children. These occur from time to time in most families. The difficulty is in deciding where to draw the line between worrying behaviour and emotional abuse. There are nevertheless characteristics of individuals, together with specific circumstances, which may make parents behave, more regularly and more extremely, in ways that will harm their children. As with other forms of abuse, emotional abuse is associated with social disadvantage. However this may reflect significant under-detection in more privileged families. Many features contributing to parenting difficulties are more common in disadvantaged families, for example teenage pregnancy, large family size, poor housing, unemployment, family breakdown and lack of social support (Browne and Saqi 1988). Psychological immaturity which can be associated with learning difficulties or personality disorder as well as chronological age, may lead to unrealistic expectations of the child's development and poor adaptation to the child's needs (Belsky and Vondra 1989).

Major risk factors in parents include alcohol and drug misuse, mental illness, learning difficulties and, in particular, personality disorders. Glaser and Prior (1997) found mental health problems including depression, manic depressive illness, schizophrenia, anorexia nervosa and suicidal behaviour in 31% of families whose children were on the child protection register for emotional abuse. In a quarter of the families domestic violence was a feature, with a similar proportion abusing drugs and/or alcohol. Doyle (1997) found, in addition to mental health problems, substance misuse and domestic violence, features that were significantly more prevalent in emotionally abusing families. These were changes of caregiver, lack of money for essentials, death of a child in the family, poor housing and large family size.

Experience of abuse and neglect in childhood make the individual more likely to develop a personality disorder and as an adult to show poor impulse control, difficulty controlling anger and to experience conflict and instability in their relationships. The parent who was in care as a child is particularly at risk if they experienced institutional care or multiple changes of placement. Oliver (1993) reviewed 60 studies and concluded that a third of children who had been abused grow up to continue a pattern of seriously inept, neglectful or abusive parenting of their own children. In addition, a further third of child victims are at risk of becoming abusive if they experience intense stress.

Effects of emotional abuse on the developing child

There are no specific effects of emotional abuse that are clearly distinguishable from other forms of abuse and neglect, in part because emotional abuse to some degree is almost always present in all forms of child abuse. It is the deviant relationship between parent and child that is mainly responsible for the enduring effects on the child's development rather than, for example, discrete episodes of sexual or physical abuse.

Attachment and the pre-school years

Effects of emotional abuse vary in relation to the form of abuse, the child's stage of development as well as specific characteristics of the child. The most important early effect is on attachment, which has profound implications for the child's future emotional and social development. Attachment research (Ainsworth et al. 1978) has formulated the classification of organized patterns of behaviour which the infant develops in relationship to his primary caregiver, originally described by Bowlby (1969). Using the 'strange situation technique' involving brief separations from their mothers, about 60% of infants are usually classified as securely attached (Group B). The remainder are anxiously attached and are either avoidant (Group A) or ambivalent (Group C). A further group of children have been identified as showing disorganized–disoriented attachment (Group D) that is associated with abusive relationships (Carlson et al. 1989).

If a child has received adequate parenting in infancy, he is securely attached to his mother or main caregiver and may be protected from some of the effects of later emotional abuse. He may show a change in behaviour or may seek out positive relationships with other adults in whom he may be able to confide, making detection and intervention more likely. In contrast the majority of abused infants are likely to be insecurely attached (Crittenden and Ainsworth 1989). They are also more likely to show the most severe type of abnormal – disorganised–disoriented – attachment, now thought to be especially associated with the child developing a fearful relationship with their main caregiver (Cicchetti and Toth 1995).

How might the health visitor or general practitioner recognize early attachment problems arising from parenting difficulties that could be emotionally abusive and require intervention? There is considerable overlap with the effects of both maternal depression and neglect. In the most extreme situation the child will fail to thrive, showing both inadequate growth as well as developmental delay. He may demonstrate avoidant attachment with behaviour such as poor eye contact, passive withdrawal or lack of social responsiveness and, later on, language delay. With anxious attachment the child may appear unusually anxious and clingy. Associated problems, such as excessive crying, severe feeding and sleeping problems, are not specific to either the parenting problem or to the type of abnormal attachment.

During the pre-school years difficulties with concentration, distractibility, severe tantrums or aggression may become more obvious, particularly in children with disorganized attachment. Some abused children between the ages of one and three years have been found to show a behaviour pattern characterized by hyper-vigilance to parental demands and quick compliance – known as 'compulsive compliance' – which contrasts with the developing autonomy and associated tantrums and challenging behaviour of normal toddlers. Disorganized attachment is particularly hard to recognize because the pattern of relating which the child shows toward his parent is so inconsistent and represents intense ambivalence.

Abnormal attachment behaviour may be difficult to detect in the relaxed atmosphere of a home visit, but behaviours associated with insecure attachment are more apparent in stressful situations. The child may avoid contact with the parent, or cry excessively following a brief separation for example. The general practitioner may observe abnormal interactions in a busy surgery. Often it is the inappropriate responses of a parent to a child's distress or challenging behaviour that alerts the professionals. This may be particularly apparent in the child health clinic when parents are waiting, dressing and undressing children and particularly managing vaccinations.

Older children

Children who are emotionally abused are likely to show increasing problems during their school years, but there are no features that are specific to this form of abuse. There is considerable overlap with emotional neglect, with children showing attention seeking behaviour, poor peer relationships, low self-esteem, aggression, poor concentration and underachievement. When children have generalized or specific learning difficulties or language delay it can be very difficult to determine whether these difficulties are constitutional or related to parenting difficulties. Some serious cases of emotional abuse or neglect go unrecognized for too long because behavioural problems are seen as secondary to learning difficulties. This is particularly likely when the parents also have learning difficulties.

Other children of apparently normal intelligence may show increasingly severe difficulties and may be at risk of exclusion from school. Their problems in the classroom and in the playground may lead to an assessment of their special educational needs. When educational interventions fail and there are no obvious explanations for enduring difficulties, emotional abuse should be considered. The strongest indicator may be the parent's attitude when the difficulties are raised with them. They may be dismissive, helpless and angry with the child or they may blame the school. Some parents deny the child shows problems at home, others may reveal they cannot cope with the child or that there is ongoing domestic violence.

Adolescents may present with any of the above problems. They may have just about coped in a good primary school because of the support and continuity of attention available, but become increasingly unmanageable after moving to secondary school where their emotional needs are less likely to be recognized or met. It is surprising how often an abusive home situation can be overlooked for many years. This can occur when the child repeatedly changes schools, perhaps moved by parents to avoid permanent exclusion or when the school begins to seek social service involvement. Sometimes the difficulties are attributed to a child's learning difficulties or poor school attendance. Truancy is particularly common. The teenager sometimes presents with a crisis which cannot be ignored so easily, an overdose, escalating violence in the home or at school, running away or involvement in criminal activities. Sometimes a young person will ask to be taken into care by social services. Unfortunately, although some new services are being developed for adolescents who are out of control it is often too little too late. Those who get caught up in the criminal justice system are particularly disadvantaged.

Characteristics of children at increased risk of emotional abuse

The children of parents who have been abused and have experienced abnormal attachments with their own parents are themselves at considerable risk of emotional abuse. Large family size increases the risk of all forms of abuse, but within an individual family some children are particularly vulnerable while others show more resilience. Children who were premature, had low birth weight or who have chronic illness, physical or intellectual handicap are at increased risk of emotional abuse. Perinatal difficulties may contribute to insecure attachment and all increase the pressures on already vulnerable overburdened parents. The visiting pattern of parents to the neonatal intensive care unit or paediatric ward, or frequent readmission to hospital in infancy for 'social' reasons or failure to thrive may alert the ward staff, and must be raised with the primary care team.

Children with difficult temperament or developmental disorders, such as specific language delay or attention deficit disorder, are particularly at risk because they are more difficult for the average parent to manage and likely to develop behaviour problems. Boys are over-represented in these groups and are also more likely to show serious behavioural problems early on as a result of emotional abuse, specifically when they witness domestic violence or experience parental hostility (Rutter and Quinton 1984). In families where the mother has experienced domestic violence, she is more likely to attribute her son's challenging behaviour to violent characteristics inherited from his father than to a reaction to the conflict he has witnessed. Thus an enduring negative view of the boy can develop which can lead to rejection, hostility, helplessness or scapegoating.

Some children appear to be less susceptible to emotional abuse. Apart from female gender, other characteristics associated with resilience are protective, high intelligence and easy sociable temperament, for example. The opportunity to form a healthy attachment is increased in these children so that when an alternative caregiver who can meet more of their emotional needs is available, albeit only temporarily, they may develop a secure attachment. This will help them to develop other positive relationships with the extended family or at school.

Recognition and assessment of emotional abuse

The difficulties for professionals involved in deciding where unsatisfactory parenting ends and emotional abuse begins have already been described. It is important to be able to identify chronic pervasive difficulties in the parent–child relationship, and to decide when intervention by social services is warranted. Except in extreme cases or when other forms of abuse have already led to the initiation of child protection procedures, emotional abuse can be more confidently identified as the core problem by the pooling of information by a number of professionals. Consistent observations of parent–child interaction over time are particularly important, as well as the views of those who are more closely involved with the child, particularly nursery staff or teachers. In these circumstances, it is advisable for the professionals involved to meet to share their observations and decide whether further assessment is necessary or whether to initiate child protection procedures. If social services are not already involved it is desirable to involve a representative at this early stage. It is good practice to inform the family that the professionals who know them will be meeting and to explain the purpose in general terms, for example to discuss how best to help the family or how to coordinate input from the professionals involved. Clearly once a decision is made to start a child protection investigation or a child in need assessment, this will need to be explained to the family who would normally be invited to any child protection conference.

Health visitors and general practitioners who have known the family for some time are especially well-placed to assist other professionals in evaluating the family situation. Sometimes they have also known the parents and their family circumstances since their childhood. Browne and Saqi (1988) showed that the observations of health visitors were particularly good predictors for identifying those families who were involved in a child protection conference concerning their pre-school children. The health visitor had made observations of parental indifference, intolerance or excessive anxiety towards the child in 84% of abusing families compared with 22% of non-abusing families. Attempts to develop checklists to identify high-risk families have met with relatively little success since other risk factors such as socio-economic disadvantage, teenage pregnancy or mental health problems are common in communities at risk. Browne and Saqi (1988) conclude that checklists may not be reliable enough to be used as screening tools for abuse. Work is currently being evaluated to see if a child-centred checklist might be useful for health visitors and social workers monitoring cases about whom there is a high level of concern, or for children on the child protection register for physical and emotional neglect (Adrian et al. 2002).

Primary care professionals are well placed to pick up concerns about domestic violence, and may be able to encourage women to reveal the extent of the problem and seek help. McGee (1999) interviewed children and their mothers who had experienced domestic violence. They found that both the mothers and the children had attended their general practitioner frequently with stress-related complaints. Once they had been able to discuss the violence, half had experienced their doctors as supportive, providing emotional and practical support, and half felt that their doctors did not want to know about the domestic violence or were too willing to prescribe tranquillizers as a solution. Although some mothers had been anxious about the possible role their health visitor could play in taking their children into care if they revealed the violence, they found them the most helpful of all professionals in terms of emotional support and practical advice about refuges and where to get help. This study, together with others, found that one third to over half of all children on the child protection register have experienced domestic violence and that most parents were unaware that their children had witnessed the violence.

Once there are serious concerns about the effects on a child of parenting difficulties, whether or not the professionals agree that child protection procedures should be initiated, it is advisable to seek an assessment from the child mental health service. It is important when making a referral to specify whether the assessment needs to be undertaken by a child psychiatrist at this stage, for example if there are likely to be legal proceedings or if the child presents a complex diagnostic problem with interacting constitutional and familial factors. It is essential to clarify the role of social services in relation to their own investigations and child protection procedures, provide details of all the professionals involved and as much information about the child's development, family background and interaction as possible. Depending on the level of concern and previous attempts to help the family, the focus of a referral may be primarily for assessment, for treatment or both, and this should be discussed with the family.

A strategic decision may be made by the professionals involved to seek a thorough assessment and/or trial of family intervention before calling a child protection conference, particularly if the family is unlikely to cooperate. Emotional abuse is probably the most difficult registration category to explain to parents. The task is facilitated with full information about the harmful effects on the child and the results of attempts to improve parenting. Obviously when parents are able to make use of support or family intervention to improve the quality of their parenting, registration may not be necessary.

Glaser and Prior (1997) reported that the mean time between the first report of concern to social services and registration for emotional abuse in 94 cases was 4 years (range 8 months to 14 years). They also noted that 78% of the children had been on the register for emotional abuse for over a year and for many there was still no clear plan for protection, either living at home or being looked after by the local authority. They go on to discuss the difficulties of using standard child protection procedures for emotional abuse because of delay in recognizing or defining it, the difficulty of monitoring an emotionally abusive relationship and the use of registration as a last resort following treatment failure before initiating legal proceedings. They recommend that child protection procedures should be used after a thorough assessment and trial of intervention over 3–6 months has failed because of lack of cooperation or insufficient change. The assessment should involve identification of parental risk factors such as mental illness, domestic violence or substance misuse, the forms of ill-treatment and the nature of the effects on the child.

Clinical example

One complex family that illustrates the difficulty in recognizing and intervening for emotional abuse, was known to the social service department from soon after the birth of the first child. The mother had mild learning difficulties and all four children had different fathers. The first and third children had significant developmental delay. The quality of care which the children received fluctuated greatly depending the contribution of two of the children's fathers and the involvement of maternal grandmother at different times. The children were first placed on the child protection register after the second son alleged that his mother's cohabitee had sexually abused him. The allegation was retracted by the boy, who was showing behavioural problems and under achieving at school. He was guarded and fiercely loyal to his mother.

Eventually the oldest boy became out of control at his special school and at home. His mother admitted she could not cope and respite care was arranged. With increased professional involvement it became apparent that his needs could not be met at home and the younger children were endangered by his aggressive behaviour towards them. A child psychiatric assessment was arranged and eventually, after improving significantly in his behaviour, learning and self-esteem in foster care, he was placed with his father on a Care Order. At this stage the father of the third child had rejoined his family and planned to marry the mother. He had a good relationship with all the children who were significantly more attached to him than to their mother. In order to give the three younger children the opportunity to remain with him and their mother, a Supervision Order was granted and further intensive input to improve the mother's parenting was arranged at a local children's centre.

Almost immediately after the care proceedings the mother left him and secretly resumed a relationship with her former cohabitee. The behaviour of all three children deteriorated markedly, and the second boy was permanently excluded from his primary school because of his extreme aggression. All three children were subsequently placed permanently in the care of the local authority although placement was problematic because of the difficulty of caring for three such disturbed children. In this case it had been the observations of the local primary care professionals of the mother's drinking, her continued and violent relationship with her cohabitee and her inconsistent limited interaction with the children, which assisted the child psychiatrist and social services in making the case for the Care Order. She was controlling, threatening and constantly critical to her second son and indifferent to her attention-seeking developmentally delayed daughter and youngest child, whom she kept in his buggy for long periods. At no time could she acknowledge any problems with her care of the children or any desire to change, although she attended the family centre regularly. All three children improved significantly with an experienced foster carer and the second son was able to disclose details of sexual abuse, his frightening aggression towards girls diminished and he began to smile. He described how care had been used as a constant threat by his mother, but he wanted to stay because it was so much better than at home.

Treatment and outcome

We know that within socially disadvantaged populations there will be many parents who are at risk of emotionally abusing their children and that for some individuals, such as mothers who were in care or abused as children, the likelihood is increased, particularly when they are socially isolated and under stress. Increasing social support and reducing stress for vulnerable parents is likely to improve the quality of their parenting. General services such as good housing, employment or adequate income, high quality nurseries, family planning, mental health services, drug and alcohol counselling, speech and language therapy and other early interventions for children with disabilities can help parents function better and provide better care for their children (Leventhal 1996). Recent programmes such as Sure Start and Education Action Zones are attempting to improve support, early intervention and accessibility of services for families with young children in deprived areas. Their effectiveness requires evaluation, but it would be difficult to demonstrate any impact on the prevalence of emotional abuse. Interventions to protect mothers and children from domestic violence, recognition and treatment for depression, drug or alcohol problems or to reduce family breakdown are likely to have more specific effects.

Once emotional abuse is recognized, as Glaser and Prior (1997) suggest, assessment and intervention should occur simultaneously. This will involve frequent direct observations of parent–child interaction, attempts to improve parenting and evaluation of the effects on the child. This may be attempted initially in an outpatient child mental health clinic or in a local family centre with staff who have been trained for this work. It may become clear that the skills or resources available locally are insufficient to undertake the intensive treatment required for some seriously disturbed individuals to change enough to avoid further significant harm to their children. Some families may be unwilling to cooperate until Children Act proceedings are initiated and they face the reality that they may lose their children. The local authority may seek an assessment at a specialist treatment unit, usually a day or residential unit with special expertise in working with families often combined with a psychodynamic approach.

In evaluating whether treatment is feasible, the assessment will consider to what extent the parents are able to recognize that their behaviour has affected their child, that they need to change and to what extent they are able to put the child's needs before their own. Do the parents continue to blame the child or the professionals and to what extent are they motivated to accept help for marital conflict, alcohol or other problems which are harming the child? The outcome of treatment will depend on their motivation and willingness to look at themselves, take feedback and demonstrate an ability to change. Jones (1987) reviewed the characteristics of 'untreatable families'. Poor outcome was associated with treatment dropouts and denial of wrongdoing. Parents with sociopathic or very inadequate personalities, persistent addiction problems or mental handicap did badly. They had often been abused as children, were hostile and showed little capacity to love or relate to others, or to empathize with the child who was regarded as a possession.

Clinical example

A seven-year-old boy was referred to the child psychiatrist by the family health visitor because his parents could not manage his behaviour and his parents thought he might have attention deficit disorder. They had previously been convinced he was autistic and would not accept the opinion of another child psychiatrist that he was not. At assessment the parents described how their son, who had been born prematurely and had asthma, had multiple behavioural problems, severe tantrums in which he hurt them and broke things, soiling with faecal smearing, nocturnal enuresis, swearing, screaming and he could not be left alone. He had mild learning difficulties but presented no problems at his special school nor during clinical interviews where he kept his head down and drew despite constant denigration by his mother.

It became apparent during intensive behavioural family therapy that his parents were completely inconsistent. They gave in to all his tantrums and indulged him indiscriminately with gifts of food and toys. He was getting increasingly overweight and his parents maintained his behaviour was getting worse. They brought tape recordings of his screaming and lists of increasing problems as they did not feel they would be believed. They could not follow advice, the father said treatment was a waste of time and when some changes were achieved they were unable to acknowledge any improvement. Although the father refused to attend further appointments the mother continued with her son and began to talk about her own abuse and ill-health as a child. She revealed her husband was drinking, spending her money and that he was like another child to care for. Eventually after a lengthy and large professionals' meeting and the persistence of the health visitor, speech therapist and child psychiatrist, social services took responsibility for the family. The children were placed on the register for emotional abuse. Only after care proceedings were initiated because social services learned from the police about severe domestic violence and that the boy had hit his father with a hammer, were the family able to follow through with referral to a specialist day unit. Although they remained anxious and lacked insight they were able follow advice, the father stopped drinking and their management of the children became more consistent. Their obvious affection and desire to parent their children well was a major factor in the improvement, coupled with consistent input from a skilled and patient social worker. The children remained at home on a Supervision Order.

In all cases the potential for treatment will need to be considered before embarking on prolonged attempts to keep the child with his parents or to rehabilitate the child from foster care. Obvious improvement in a younger child once placed in foster care, or persistence of severe disturbance in an older child making them difficult to care for, are important indicators that the relationship with the parent was sufficiently damaging to warrant consideration of permanent removal of the child. In the sample of children on the child protection register for emotional abuse followed up by Glaser and Prior (1997), a third were permanently removed and a third remained with their parents, who were more likely to have been able to acknowledge the emotional abuse. One third remained at home or in care while interventions were continuing.

Trowell *et al.* (1997) described intensive psychodynamic family work in a day unit and Stevenson (1999) reviewed a wide variety of treatments. They both concluded that parenting can be changed with training but that treatment needs to be provided over long periods. Successful treatment will have an impact on parental functioning as well as that of the child, although the parent may still view the child negatively. When children are placed permanently away from their parents they will usually require treatment, behaviour therapy to help their carers or school to manage their behaviour and individual psychotherapy where available as well as support for the carers.

General practitioners and health visitors can play key roles in the recognition, assessment and treatment of emotional abuse because of their long-term relationships with families. They will rarely need to use the term emotional abuse directly with families, but careful recording of their observations over time and referrals at the appropriate stage to social services or to child mental health services are crucial in the management of this challenging problem. Observations of interactions in the surgery or at home, as well as those of practice staff e.g. receptionists, will continue to assist social services during assessment and a trial of intervention. It can be difficult for the GP to balance the need to maintain a therapeutic alliance with a vulnerable parent and the need to protect the child. Fortunately, decisions about permanent removal of children are usually made relatively late by social services after input from a number of professionals. Meanwhile the recognition of less severe parenting difficulties and referral for support and treatment is likely to have a beneficial impact on a large number of children and will be appreciated by the majority of parents.

References

Adrian N, Hall A, Harris R and Gold J (2002) When is it neglect? The development of a tool to record and monitor features associated with the neglect of children. *Report for Tower Hamlets Area Child Protection Committee.*

Ainsworth M, Blehar M, Waters E and Wall S (1978) *Patterns of Attachment.* Hillsdale, NJ: Lawrence Erlbaum Associates.

Belsky J and Vondra J (1989) Lessons from child abuse: the determinants of parenting, in D Cicchetti, V Carlson (eds) *Child Maltreatment: Theory and Research on the Causes and Consequences of Child Abuse and Neglect.* New York: Cambridge University Press.

Bowlby J (1969) *Attachment and Loss. Vol. 1: Attachment.* New York: Basic Books.

Browne K and Saqi S (1988) Approaches to screening for child abuse and neglect, in K Browne, C Davies, P Stratton (eds) *Early Prediction and Prevention of Child Abuse.* Chichester: John Wiley.

Carlson V, Cicchetti D, Barnett D and Braunwald K (1989) Disorganised/disoriented attachment relationships in maltreated infants. *Developmental Psychopathology* 25: 163–73.

Cicchetti D (ed.) (1991) Special issue: defining psychological maltreatment. *Development and Psychopathology* 3(1).

Cicchetti D and Toth S (1995) Child maltreatment and attachment organisation: implications for intervention, in S Goldberg, R Muir, J Kerr (eds) *Attachment Theory: Social, Developmental and Clinical Perspectives.* Hillsdale, NJ: Analytic Press.

Crittenden PM and Ainsworth MDS (1989) Child maltreatment and attachment theory, in D Cicchetti, V Carlson (eds) *Child Maltreatment: Theory and Research on the Causes and Consequences of Child Abuse and Neglect.* New York: Cambridge University Press.

Crowe HP and Zeskind PS (1992) Psychophysiological and perceptual responses to infant cries varying in pitch: comparison of adults with high and low scores on the child abuse potential inventory. *Child Abuse and Neglect* 16: 19–29.

Department of Health (1988) *Protecting Children: A Guide for Social Workers Undertaking a Comprehensive Assessment.* London: HMSO.

Department of Health, Home Office, Department for Education and Employment (1999) *Working Together to Safeguard Children: A Guide to Inter-agency Working to Safeguard and Promote the Welfare of Children*. London: HMSO.

Doyle C (1997) Emotional abuse of children: issues for intervention. *Child Abuse Review* 6: 330–42.

Fogarty M (1980) Emotional abuse to be included in registers. *Social Work Today* 12(1): 4.

Gabarino J, Guttman E and Seeley J (1986) *The Psychologically Battered Child*. San Francisco: Jossey-Bass.

Glaser D (1993) Emotional abuse, in CJ Hobbs, JM Wynne, JES Fortin (eds) *Clinical Paediatric, International Practice and Research: Child Abuse* 1:1 London: Balliere Tindall.

Glaser D and Prior V (1997) Is the term child protection applicable to emotional abuse? *Child Abuse Review* 6: 315–29.

Hart SN and Brassard MR (1987) A major threat to children's mental health: psychological maltreatment. *American Psychologist* 41: 160–5.

Jones DPH (1987) The untreatable family. *Child Abuse and Neglect*. 11: 409–20.

Leventhal JM (1996) Twenty years later: we do know how to prevent child abuse and neglect. *Child Abuse and Neglect* 20: 647–55.

McGee C. (1999) *Childhood Experiences of Domestic Violence*. London: Jessica Kingsley Publishers.

McGee RA and Wolfe DA (1991) Psychological maltreatment: toward an operational definition. *Development and Psychopathology* 3(1): 3–18.

Oliver JE (1993) Intergenerational transmission of child abuse: rates, research and clinical implications. *American Journal of Psychiatry* 150: 1315–24.

Patterson GR, DeBaryshe BD and Ramsay E (1989) A developmental perspective on antisocial behaviour. *American Psychologist* 44: 329–35.

Pynoos RS and Eth S (1986) Witness to violence: the child interview. *Journal of the American Academy of Child and Adolescent Psychiatry* 25: 306–19.

Rushton A (2000) Psychological perspectives on the impact of domestic violence on children. Conference proceedings: *Domestic Violence: Lifelong Consequences*. Liverpool: Liverpool University Law School.

Rutter M and Quinton D (1984) Parental psychiatric disorder: effects on children. *Psychological Medicine* 14: 853–80.

Skuse D and Bentovim A (1994) Physical and emotional maltreatment, in M Rutter, E Taylor, L Hersov (eds) *Child and Adolescent Psychiatry: Modern Approaches*. Oxford: Blackwell Scientific.

Stevenson J (1999) The treatment of the long term sequelae of child abuse. *Journal of Child Psychology and Psychiatry* 40(1): 89–111.

Thompson AE and Kaplan CA (1996) Childhood emotional abuse. *British Journal of Psychiatry* 168: 143–8.

Trowell J, Hodges S and Leighton-Laing J (1997) Emotional abuse: the work of a family centre. *Child Abuse Review* 6: 357–69.

Chapter 9

Child sexual abuse

Alison Mott

Introduction

General practitioners and health visitors, as a result of their close relationship with families in their communities, have an important role to play in the diagnosis and initial management of the child who has been sexually abused. Since the child and alleged perpetrator may both be registered with the practice, suspicion of abuse has to be handled carefully and it may be difficult to judge when concerns about abuse are sufficient for action to be taken. However, all members of the primary health care team are legally and ethically required to report all types of suspected abuse. General practitioners are not responsible for making the diagnosis of sexual abuse, but are obliged to identify children suspected of being abused and to refer them to social services. In this chapter, I will describe:

+ Some of the ways in which sexual abuse may present; (Table 9.1)
+ The general practitioner's role in the initial management;
+ How the diagnosis of abuse is confirmed.

Definition

Child sexual abuse is defined as the sexual exploitation of a child for the gratification of an adult. Children of all ages are abused, including infants. Boys and girls are abused, but boys are less likely to report the abuse or to be believed when they make disclosures. Sexual abuse of children involves many types of sexual activities, from non-contact activities such as flashing or pornography to contact activities including touching and violent rape. Sexual activities should only occur between consenting persons, and children are unable to make an informed decision. However, sexual exploratory play between children of similar ages is a normal part of development. For teenagers, it may be difficult to judge whether they are consenting to sexual activities. For example, a 14-year-old girl can have sufficient understanding to consent to sexual activities with an older person. However if coercion or force is used, a different interpretation is needed.

Table 9.1 Presentation of child sexual abuse (Vizard and Tranter 1988)

Disclosure	By child or third party
Physical indicators	Rectal or vaginal bleeding, pain on defaecation Sexually transmitted disease (STD) Vulvovaginitis/vaginal discharge/ 'sore' Dysuria and frequency ?UTI Physical abuse, note association of burns, pattern of injury, death Pregnancy
Psychosomatic indicators	Recurrent abdominal pain Headache, migraine Anorexia or other eating disorders Encopresis Enuresis Total refusal syndrome
Behavioural indicators: (i) Pre-school	Sexually explicit play 'Excessive' masturbation Insertion of foreign bodies Self mutilation Withdrawn Poor appetite Sleep disturbance Clingy Delayed development Aggression
(ii) Middle years	Sexualized play Sexually explicit drawing or sexual precocity Self-mutilation Anxiety and depression Anger Poor school performance Mute
(iii) Teenagers	Sexually precocious Prostitution Anxiety, anger, aggression, depression Truancy, running away Solvent/alcohol/drug abuse Self-destructive behaviour, overdoses, self-mutilation, suicide
Learning difficulties/physical disability	May present with depression, disturbed behaviour Sexualized behaviour Attempts at disclosure not understood May be physical and psychosomatic indicators as above
Social indicators	Concern by parent or third party, sibling, relative or friend of abused child Schedule 1 offender in close contact with child

Incidence of sexual abuse

The incidence of sexual abuse is 1.5–3 times higher in females than males. Surveys from the adult general population indicate that 7–36% of females and 3–29% of males were abused as children (Finkelhor 1994). The wide range in incidence in epidemiological studies is dependant on the definition of sexual abuse used, the questions asked and the survey methodology. The UK rates in a MORI 1985 study were 12% for females and 8% for males (Baker and Duncan 1985). This was half the incidence found in an American study in which more sensitive questions were asked. The rates reported by adults are significantly higher than the level of reported cases in children, since sexual abuse is under-recognized in childhood.

A postal survey in Scotland in 1992 showed that 73% of GPs had seen at least one case of sexual abuse in the last 2 years (Bisset and Hunter 1992). This indicates an incidence of 2.5 cases per 1000 per year for girls aged under 16 years in general practice and of 0.8 per 1000 per year for boys aged under 12 years. Although the incidence may vary from area to area, abuse can occur in all communities and in families of any background. Thus all general practitioners will encounter sexually abused children.

Patterns of abuse

Sexual abuse often occurs against a background of other family problems, and is linked with other categories of abuse and neglect. Child sexual abuse can be intra-familial, extrafamilial, institutional or stranger abuse. In the majority of cases the child knows the abuser, either as a family member, friend of the family or person in a position of power over the child. Sexual assaults on children by strangers are rare, although this is not currently well understood by the tabloid press. Abusers include both men and women. Another child or adolescent may also sexually abuse a child. For example, 25% of children abused in a study in Leeds were abused by teenagers (Hobbs *et al.* 1999). Many of the abusers have been sexually abused themselves and the majority have had impoverished childhoods.

Abusers groom children over a long period of time. The child develops an adjustment pattern to the abuse, known as the *Accommodation syndrome*. The characteristics of the syndrome are secrecy, helplessness, accommodation, delayed disclosure and retraction. Thus children keep silent, are unable to stop the abuse, blame themselves, don't disclose or if they do, retract the disclosure, even when subject to long-term abuse. Children rarely fabricate disclosures of sexual abuse and inconsistencies in their story do not imply that the child has lied. However, unfortunately, these inconsistencies can make prosecution of the abuser difficult.

Effects of sexual abuse

Child sexual abuse has enormous impact on the health of our society. Short-term effects include behavioural problems, school failure and difficulties forming friendships. If abuse has occurred in a significant relationship, for example with a parent, the child will find it difficult to establish trusting relationships. Long-term effects are mental health problems, sexual relationship difficulties and social dysfunction. The effects may last into the victim's relationship with their own children. Adults who have been sexually abused as children may present to general practitioners and adult mental health services.

Recognition and clinical presentation

Members of the primary health care team will never identify children who have been abused without a willingness to consider the possibility of sexual abuse. This can be difficult for health professionals, who may have known the family for some time, and who may believe that 'it couldn't happen in a family like that'. A high index of suspicion is required, and health professionals have to acknowledge that child sexual abuse can occur in any family.

A further aspect to recognition is having confidence in the child protection process once referral has been made. If a professional lacks confidence about the quality of response that will occur, she may feel that it is easier not to think about sexual abuse and avoid referral. There has been very little research on the clinical presentation of sexual abuse to general practitioners or other members of the primary health care team. Often they only become involved when they are informed by the Community Paediatrician or by the Social Worker investigating the case. However, children may present directly in a variety of ways that raise the possibility of sexual abuse and indicate a need for referral.

A 12-year-old girl discloses to her mother that the lodger has been trying to kiss her and touch her pants. The mother attends surgery, as she doesn't know what to do.
The GP needs to tell the mother that immediate referral to Social Services is needed. It is important to establish time of last contact as this can influence the timing of the examination.

The commonest clinical presentation of sexual abuse is disclosure by the child. This can be to a family member, a friend or a professional such as teacher, family planning nurse or general practitioner. When a disclosure is made, it is important to acknowledge what has been said, and inform the child that you will have to pass this information onto the relevant professionals within social services. You may have to clarify simple details before referral, but it is important not to interrogate the child about the disclosure as this could affect the evidence from a legal perspective. If a child asks you not to tell anyone else, it is important to be honest and say it is for the protection of her and other children.

Another person may be concerned that a child is being abused, for example a parent, relative or friend. Alternatively, you may be informed that a Schedule 1 offender, a person convicted of crime against children, has moved into the house of a child about whom you have other concerns. Disclosure by a child is not necessary for formal investigation to take place.

A 13-year-old girl, who has just been found to be pregnant, does not want her parents to know. She is reluctant to tell you who the father is.
There are many issues here but sexual abuse must be considered. A discussion with Social Services would be essential.

Clear physical indicators include pregnancy, sexually transmitted disease and rectal bleeding (Vizard and Tranter 1988). All pre-pubertal girls with vaginal bleeding need referral. Other symptoms such as vulval soreness, vaginal discharge, or urinary symptoms of dysuria and frequency without a urinary tract infection need assessment in the light of the overall context of the presentation.

The mother of a 4-year-old girl tells you that her daughter has a sore itchy bottom, following a weekend stay with her ex-husband, the father of the child. She is concerned that he has been sexually abusing her. Access issues are currently being contested in court.
As the mother is raising the possibility of sexual abuse, again the family needs to be immediately referred to Social Services. The child protection investigation will have to assess the issues around contested access.

Psychosomatic indicators in both boys and girls are recurrent abdominal pain, headaches, anorexia, enuresis and encopresis. Behavioural symptoms vary with the age of the child and include abnormal sexual behaviour, withdrawal, delayed development, poor school attendance and drug and alcohol misuse. It must be remembered that there is a strong overlap in the clinical presentation of physical and sexual abuse. Patterns of physical injury, which suggest that sexual abuse may also have occurred, include grip marks on upper arms and thighs and bruises on lower abdomen.

Alternatively children may be asymptomatic or simply not present to the primary health care team. A study from Wales found that in 107 boys abused by their primary school teacher, none had disclosed abuse to their GP (Maddocks *et al.* 1999). Only two had presented with any symptoms at the time, but neither was identified as sexual abuse. There was no difference in the frequency of behavioural or somatic symptoms between these children and a similar sample of non-abused control children. The only significant finding was that the symptoms persisted longer in the abused boys, both at 3 months and at 1 year. The recommendation was that GPs must keep an open mind about the possibility of sexual abuse in boys who had persistent and inexplicable symptoms over a long period. Careful questioning by practitioners might encourage further disclosure.

What do you do with a girl with vaginal discharge?

A 6-year-old girl has recurrent vaginal discharge. Vaginal swabs taken in surgery have shown growths of streptococci. Despite treatment the discharge is becoming increasingly offensive and the mother and child attend surgery wanting help. The girl has some small red haemorrhagic bruises on her vulva.

What do you do with a girl with vaginal discharge? *(continued)*

The possibility of sexual abuse should always be considered when a child presents with genital symptoms, particularly if these are persistent. Referral must always be made to either a clinician or Social Services.

The management of vaginal discharge in pre-pubertal girls presents particular difficulty. A high proportion of girls who have been sexually abused have vulvitis or vulvovaginitis. However, only a small proportion of girls with vulvovaginitis have been sexually abused. Therefore child sexual abuse needs to be considered but in clinical practice is rare. Vulvovaginitis can be due to hormonal and physical reasons. It is reasonable for initial management to be conservative with simple advice regarding cotton pants, loose clothing, soaking in daily baths, and avoidance of irritants in the bath. Threadworms should be considered and treated. Anti-fungal creams are usually unhelpful as fungal infection is rare except after antibiotics therapy.

Antibiotics should not be prescribed without investigation. However, the clinician should consider the possibility of sexual abuse before taking a swab. The parents should be asked if they have any particular concerns related to the cause of the discharge that they want to discuss. It is important not to upset the child or even cause injury, particularly if a further examination is needed. A swab of profuse discharge may be taken if the labia are parted and a moistened swab placed gently between them. The swab should not be inserted into the vagina.

Interpretation of the results needs to be undertaken with care. It may be assumed that the presence of an organism on bacteriological culture indicates the cause of the symptoms. However, a recent case control study of children with vulvovaginitis found that both cases and controls had similar microbiology (Jaquiery *et al.* 1999). Infections of streptococci or staphylococci may be treated with the appropriate antibiotics. However, if evidence of a sexually transmitted disease is found immediate referral should be made to the child protection investigation team, including a paediatrician.

Recurrent episodes of discharge or persistent symptoms after treatment need referral to a paediatrician or gynaecologist with a special interest in paediatric gynaecology for a full assessment.

What should the primary care team do?

The Health Visitor discusses a child at the practice meeting. She is worried about the sexualized behaviour of a 3-year-old girl. She is using inappropriate sexual vocabulary and is playing sexual games with her dolls. There have been no other concerns about the family in the practice.

This case presents a challenge, as it may be difficult to assess whether there is enough information to refer the child. If there is any concern about child sexual abuse it is important to share this information with Social Services. They may discover further information, for example that the mother's new boyfriend is a Schedule 1 offender. It is possible to discuss children with Social Services and not inform the family, as this could warn the abuser.

The diagnosis of child abuse has been compared to a jigsaw: the different pieces of information need to be put together to get the full picture. If a general practitioner suspects sexual abuse, she must pass this information on. Discussion between the primary care team can be helpful. All referrals should be made to Social Services, although this may follow discussion with the local Community Paediatrician. Social Services will carefully consider the information and may be aware of other concerns about the family, which have previously been insufficient to act upon.

General practitioners may be concerned about breaching patient confidentiality. However, GMC guidelines state that if you suspect or believe a child to be a victim of sexual abuse, you should give information promptly to a statutory agency. If for any reason you believe this is not in the child's best interests and do not refer, you must be able to justify this decision. The Children's Act 1989 clearly puts the welfare of the child first, and this supports referral to statutory agencies even when other members of the family who are patients of the general practitioner are being incriminated.

Where appropriate, those with parental responsibility for the victim should be informed. However, this may not be straightforward. Suspicion of abuse is likely to raise considerable emotions within the victim's family and the issue must be treated sensitively and with the provision of considerable support. If the abuse is intrafamilial, warning the abuser of the referral gives him the opportunity to manipulate and control the child, who may withdraw the allegation. It also allows removal of any forensic evidence. Therefore, informing the family depends on the presentation of the child and the consent of the parents is not required before referral. If there is any concern that the abuser might be warned, the family should not be told of the referral.

It is very important to keep accurate contemporaneous notes and record all your actions, including telephone calls to other professionals. If a disclosure is made, you should write down everything the child says in her own words. You should assume that all cases are going to court, usually in some months time, and that you will have to report and justify your actions (or the lack of them).

All general practitioners and health visitors should understand their local Child Protection Procedures and the actions to be taken if an abused child presents. For example, in Cardiff, there is a Child Protection Emergency Team that takes all acute referrals including child sexual abuse. If there is uncertainty about the need for referral it can be very useful to talk to experienced social workers who can provide guidance on what action should be taken. Close working relationships between the professional groups involved can reduce the inevitable concerns about triggering a formal Child Protection investigation. Community Paediatricians also have expertise in the diagnosis of sexual abuse and should be available to discuss the management of cases or suspected cases of abuse.

Child protection investigation

Following a referral to Social Services of a child who may have been abused, a child protection investigation occurs. It may be that after a few simple inquiries, no further action is taken. However, if the concerns remain, the family and child will be interviewed. The child is interviewed by experienced police and social workers and is encouraged to tell her story in her own words. This interview is video-recorded and the video is used by the Crown Prosecution Service to determine the quality of evidence and the child's ability to be a witness. If the alleged abuser is charged, the video can be used in court. Unfortunately the child will still be cross-examined in court, but usually via a videolink in another room. Social services have a responsibility to inform the referrer of the outcome of the investigation. Following the disclosure interview, the child will have a medical examination by an experienced paediatrician.

Medical assessment by paediatrician

The medical assessment is part of the child protection investigation. Even if the child has only disclosed being touched, a formal paediatric assessment and examination should occur. The child may not have fully disclosed the extent of the abuse and the paediatrician may identify other health problems, such as growth delay or failure to thrive.

The purpose of the examination is to:

+ examine the child for clinical signs of abuse
+ screen children for sexually transmitted disease and pregnancy where indicated
+ treat medical problems as needed
+ take forensic evidence to support the child's disclosure
+ reassure the child and family that there is no lasting physical damage
+ identify psychological and emotional support for the child.

An experienced paediatrician, in the presence of a nurse or chaperone in a child friendly environment, should perform the examination. No doctor should undertake the formal assessment of a child unless they are familiar with the range of physical signs that are indicative of sexual abuse (Royal College of Physicians of London 1997). Facilities are needed for screening for sexually transmitted diseases, including secure transport mechanisms to maintain the chain of evidence. The timing of the examination is important if forensic evidence may be present. If the suspected contact or assault has occurred in the last 6 days, examination should be carried out as soon as possible since spermatozoa can survive up to 6 days in the vagina. Forensic evidence will be sought as part of the assessment and if found will play a vital part in the legal process. DNA sampling methods are becoming increasingly sophisticated and may lead to the abuser pleading guilty; thus the child avoids going to court.

The aim is to examine the child once and therefore in the best circumstances. Repeat examinations are only done where clinically indicated. Some centres now use a colposcope that enables a well-illuminated, magnified view of the genitalia with the facility for taking photographs or videos. If there is difficulty in interpreting clinical signs, the photographs can be discussed with colleagues and can provide evidence in the court case. It is very important that the examination is not seen as further abuse to the child. The majority of children have no difficulties with the examination. Rarely, examination under general anaesthetic will be needed when there is a high likelihood of significant medical findings. The presence of signs depends on the timing of the examination and the type of abuse. The signs are interpreted as being either diagnostic of penetrating injury or not diagnostic but supportive of abuse (Royal College of Physicians 1997). In the majority of children examined for suspected child sexual abuse, no physical findings are present and the examination may be normal, even in cases of abusive penetrative intercourse in a young child. Thus it is very important to appreciate that the absence of signs does not indicate that the child has not been abused.

Sexually transmitted diseases

A 2-year-old girl presents to your surgery with blood in her pants. The only explanation mother can suggest is that she fell over backwards over a sack of potatoes. On examination of the child's genitalia, you think you can see warts.

Current literature suggests that 50% of children with warts have been sexually abused. Therefore all children presenting with anogenital warts need to be referred for a medical assessment and to be screened for other sexually transmitted diseases.

The prevalence of sexually transmitted diseases (STD) in sexually abused children varies with the prevalence of these diseases in the abusing population (Robinson 1998; Hammerschlag 1998). The prevalence in children who have been sexually abused is 2–7% for girls and 0–5% for boys. The commonest infections are gonorrhoea, genital warts and chlamydia. Isolation of a sexually transmitted organism may be the first indication that abuse has occurred. However the majority of STDs are asymptomatic and are only identified as part of the medical examination when swabs are routinely taken. The relationship of STD and sexual abuse is complex and varies with each organism. Transmission may be perinatal or sexual or non-sexual contact. Gonorrhea in a child aged over 12 months is strongly associated with abuse. Vaginal infection is usually symptomatic but pharyngeal and rectal is not. Chlamydia trachomatis genital infection is usually asymptomatic. Perinatally acquired infection may persist for up to 3 years, but after this it is strongly suggestive of abuse. Sexually active adolescents have the highest rates of infection and are at serious risk of sequelae such as pelvic inflammatory disease.

Trichomonas vaginalis in a child over 12 months suggests recent sexual contact and is usually symptomatic. Bacterial vaginosis is a polymicrobial infection causing vaginal discharge. It is uncommon in healthy non-abused children and may be acquired after sexual abuse, but it does not provide strong evidence. It can be the cause of chronic vaginal discharge in children.

The role of human papilloma virus causing anogenital warts is unclear in relation to sexual abuse (Atabaki and Paradise 1999). Children with anogenital warts (AGW) need to be properly screened for other STD. Current literature suggests that 50% of children with AGW have been sexually abused. AGW in a child less than 3 years is probably secondary to perinatal acquisition, over 3 years sexual contact is the most likely source. The mother of the child also needs screening: 52% of mothers of 42 children with AGW had cervical intraepithelial neoplasia.

Herpes simplex infection presents as vesicular or ulcerated painful genital lesions with lymphadenopathy. It is possible to link the type of infection between the child and the perpetrator, thus providing strong evidence.

Human immunodeficiency virus (HIV) is rare but sexual abuse is a possible source. Hepatitis B and hepatitis C also need to be considered. Screening for HIV should only be undertaken after counselling the child and family, as positive results have enormous implications for the child and potentially the mother.

Post coital contraception

Post menarcheal girls presenting within 72 hours of an acute episode of abuse should be offered emergency contraception. If the incident has occurred between 72 hours and 5 days of presentation they can be offered an emergency IUD, although this would need discussion with the girl regarding the risk of infection. If there is longer delay in presentation then pregnancy testing must be undertaken.

Inter-agency communication

Inter-agency communication is key to the child protection investigation and ongoing management of the child. Members of the primary health care team have a vital role as they have an established relationship with the family. They have a responsibility to share information with other agencies should concerns about sexual abuse arise. Following the child sexual abuse investigation, decisions need to be taken on further action. This includes prosecution of the alleged abuser and ensuring the safety of the child.

Social workers have a specific role in protecting the child. The child's safety will depend on the identity of the abuser and the reaction within the family. All children need support through the child protection process but it can be particularly difficult if the family does not believe the child. This can occur if the alleged assailant is the mother's partner and she chooses to believe the partner rather than the child. If there are concerns regarding the child's safety at home, a case conference will be arranged. It is very important that key people attend the conference or at least provide a report, and often the general practitioner or health visitor has a unique contribution to make.

The role of the police is to investigate if there is a case for prosecution. They will take statements from all involved in the case, prepare a report and present it to the Crown Prosecution Service.

Ongoing management of child and family

Protection from further abuse is the first essential task for those caring for the child. Referral to child and adolescent mental health needs to be considered for each child. Support for the child and family is needed. The abused child's parents, especially the non-abusive carer, face major stress and may have considerable psychological needs, both during and after the child protection investigation. Parent's needs are often put secondary to the child's, yet meeting the needs of the parents is associated with a better outcome for the child. Therefore it is important to work with the parents as well as the child and provide adequate support.

Summary of primary care team role

Health professionals have to recognize that child sexual abuse occurs within their practice (Guidry 1995). Acknowledging this allows them to recognize the many and varied clinical presentations of child sexual abuse. Disclosure to friends, family or trusted professionals is the commonest presentation. However, signs associated with sexual abuse such as change in behaviour, abdominal pains and recurrent vaginal discharge in children commonly present to the primary health care team. Each presentation needs careful consideration with a high index of suspicion of sexual abuse.

The primary health care team is in a unique position with their knowledge of that family. They are aware of changes in the family structure and clinical presentation. However they cannot dismiss the possibility of sexual abuse, even if they have no previous concerns. A low threshold of referral to Social Services is required. Advice can be sort from the local Social Services regarding a professional's concerns. Community paediatricians are also in a position to offer advice or assessment of the child. Close working inter-agency relationships is important in the child protection process and enable early referral, prompt assessment and informed decision-making. The diagnosis of child sexual abuse is complex, involving piecing together all available information. Assessment of the child in relation to sexual abuse is multiagency, in particular involving Social Services, the police and health. The medical assessment needs to be done by a paediatrician experienced in the interpretation of clinical signs with facilities for investigation. Medical evidence can be supportive or diagnostic, but more commonly clinical examination is normal. The legal processes have inappropriately high expectations of the medical evidence. The most important piece of information is the disclosure by the child.

When children present to their GP with symptoms associated with sexual abuse such as recurrent vaginal discharge and anogenital warts, referral of the child to the appropriate specialist is needed for full assessment.

References

Atabaki S and Paradise JE (1999) The medical evaluation of the sexually abused child: lessons from a decade of research. *Pediatrics* 104(1): 178–86.

Bisset A and Hunter D (1992) Child sexual abuse in general practice in north east Scotland. *Health Bulletin* 50(3): 237–47.

Finkelhor D (1994) The international epidemiology of child sexual abuse. *Child Abuse and Neglect* 18(5): 409–17.

Guidry HM (1995) Childhood sexual abuse: Role of the family physician. *American Family Physician* 51(2): 407–18.

Hammerschlag MR (1998) Sexually transmitted diseases in sexually abused children: medical and legal implications. *Sexually Transmitted Infection* 74: 167–74.

Hobbs CJ, Hanks HGI and Wynne JM (1999) *Child Abuse and Neglect: A Clinician's Handbook.* London: Churchill Livingstone.

Jaquiery A, Stylianopoulos A, Hogg G and Grover S (1999) Vulvovaginitis: clinical features, aetiology, and microbiology of the genital tract. *Archives of Disease in Childhood* 81(1): 64–7.

Maddocks A, Griffiths L and Antao V (1999) Detecting child sexual abuse in general practice: a retrospective case-control study from Wales. *Scandinavian Journal of Primary Health Care* 17: 210–14.

Robinson AJ (1998) Sexually transmitted organisms in children and child sexual abuse. *International Journal of STD and AIDS* 9: 501–11.

Royal College of Physicians of London (1997) *Physical Signs of Sexual Abuse in Children.* London: Royal College of Physicians of London.

Vizard E and Tranter M (1988) Recognition and assessment of sexual abuse, in A Bentovim *et al.* (eds) *Child Sexual Abuse Within the Family.* London: Wright.

Further reading

Baker AW and Duncan SP (1985) Child sexual abuse: a study of prevalence in Great Britain. *Child Abuse and Neglect* 9: 457–67.

Hobbs CJ, Hanks HGI and Wynne JM (1999) *Child Abuse and Neglect: A Clinician's Handbook.* London: Churchill Livingstone.

Heger A and Emans SJ (1992) *Evaluation of the Sexually Abused Child. A Medical Textbook and Photographic Atlas.* Oxford: Oxford University Press.

General Medical Council (2000) *Confidentiality and Providing Information.* London: General Medical Council.

Jones DPH and Ramchandani P (1999) *Child Sexual Abuse: Informing Practice from Research.* Oxford: Radcliffe Medical Press.

Chapter 10

Forgotten patients – adults abused as children

Christopher Cloke

The recognition of child abuse, especially child sexual abuse, and the development of professional responses, have occurred comparatively recently. Physical abuse and the battered baby syndrome were first identified in the 1960s. Child sexual abuse shot to prominence in the late 1980s, particularly at the time of the Cleveland cases. More recently consideration has been given to the phenomenon of 'organized abuse'. Over the last two decades (1980–2000) guidance for professionals working with children who are at risk or who have been abused has been issued by government and the appropriate professional bodies. Recognition of and responses to the needs of *adults* who were abused as children has lagged a long way behind meeting the needs of children who have been abused. This is a very serious omission, since it is known that child abuse can have very damaging long term consequences, affecting both emotional and physical well being.

In the course of their work general practitioners and primary health care teams are likely to encounter a significant number of adults who were abused as children and who, as a result of the harm they suffered then, are experiencing difficulties and ill health now. The origins of these patients' ill health or lack of well being may be masked or concealed. They may be reluctant to disclose their childhood abuse for a variety of reasons – not least because of the stigma attached to having been abused and fears that they will not be believed. General practitioners and other primary care workers, in comparison with other professional groups, are considered to be accessible and adult survivors may turn to them for help. The experience of this group of patients is that the response they receive is often found to be lacking.

There has been little research into how many adults who were abused as children are to be found in the population served by a typical general practice. One study suggests that 7–9 adult survivors per 1,000 patients is likely (Pearce and Smith 1994).

Most victims of abuse tell no one at the time

The National Commission of Inquiry into the Prevention of Child Abuse took written evidence, mostly in the form of letters, from over 1000 members of the public, the large majority of whom had experienced child abuse themselves or had a close relationship with someone who had (National Commission of Inquiry into the Prevention of Child Abuse 1996). Many of these people wrote with passion and at great length. For a great number the effects of child abuse had been traumatic and lasting. Together this collection of accounts represents the largest sample of adult survivors' experiences ever brought together in the United Kingdom, and it yields a wealth of information. This was analysed for the Commission by Wattam and Woodward (1996) who particularly highlighted the lack of reporting of abuse both in childhood and in adulthood.

Only 32% of the adults writing to the Commission had told someone about the abuse they experienced while they were children: 31% had told someone as an adult and 13% has never told anyone. From this it can be seen that while a significant number of adults will disclose their childhood abuse in adulthood, a large number never tell anybody. Some will be living with significant distress and ill health (Wattam and Woodward 1996).

Research conducted by the NSPCC into the prevalence of child maltreatment found similarly high levels of under-reporting. The NSPCC study provides authoritative data on the prevalence of child abuse (Cawson *et al.* 2000). It substantiates the need to prevent child abuse and provide services and support to adults who were abused as children. The research asked a nationally representative sample of 2,869 adults aged 18–24 about their childhood experiences and it found that while nine out of ten young people said that they had warm and loving backgrounds, significant minorities had suffered serious abuse or neglect.

- Physical abuse – 7% suffered serious physical abuse as children at the hands of parents and carers. This was defined as violence causing injury or occurring regularly throughout childhood, and usually causing pain or marks lasting at least until the next day. A quarter of the respondents had experienced physical violence by being beaten with an implement, punched, kicked, knocked down, choked, burned, scalded or severely shaken at least on one occasion, usually at home, and at the hands of their birth parents.

- Neglect – 6% suffered serious physical neglect at home, including being left regularly without food as a young child, not being looked after or taken to the doctor when ill, or being left to fend for themselves because parents were absent or had drug or alcohol problems. Five per cent had been placed at risk by being left alone at home overnight or out overnight, with their whereabouts unknown, at young ages.

- Emotional abuse – 6% had suffered multiple attacks on their emotional well-being and self-confidence, including living with frequent violence between parents, being 'really afraid' of parents, being regularly humiliated, being threatened with being sent away or thrown out, or being told that their parents wished them dead or never born.

- Sexual abuse – 1% had been sexually abused by a parent and 3% suffered sexual abuse by another relative, ranging from penetrative or oral sex to taking pornographic photographs of them. One in ten – mostly girls – had been forced into sex acts against their will by people known to them under the age of sixteen.

A number of the findings of the *Child Maltreatment Study* have implications for our understanding of the needs of adults who were abused as children, and the appropriate professional responses.

- The under-reporting of child abuse. While there are around 30,000 children on child protection registers at any one time, the *Child Maltreatment Study* indicates that registrations represent only a small proportion of the children and young people who are at risk of cruelty and neglect.

- Children and young people find it difficult to talk about their experiences. In all, one in four young people said there were things that happened to them during their childhood that they found difficult to talk about. Only just over a quarter of respondents who had been sexually abused or coerced into sexually activity had told anyone at the time. One in three has *never* told anyone. This not only high-lights the need to make it easier for children to tell about their experiences, but indicates that there are many adults who are still facing difficulties and distress.

- Hardly any of the young people had told social services, teachers, police or other professionals about their experiences. Friends and relatives were the usual confi-dantes. This highlights the need to provide services that are confidential, accessible and perceived as supportive. If the victims of abuse felt this when they were young it is likely that they hold similar views in adulthood.

While the NSPCC study of child maltreatment interviewed a representative group of all 18–21 year olds who had a postal address, the methodology excluded an important group of young people – those with no fixed address. That group includes those young people who are living on the streets or 'drifting around' and a sizeable number of care-leavers. A significant proportion of those people will have come from abusive backgrounds, both in their family homes and in residential institutions. The NSPCC has estimated that care leavers are 50 times more likely to go to prison, 60 times more likely to be homeless, and 88 times more likely to take drugs than other young people. A survey by the *Big Issue* magazine found that 22% of their vendors said they has been abused as a child or adolescent and over a third of vendors have not had a place to call their own since their teens. Reaching this group of young people and adults poses particular challenges to health care teams.

The NSPCC study of child maltreatment confirms many of the National Com-mission's findings, based on the letters it received from adults who were abused as children. Wattam and Woodward found that those who told as children were more likely to be younger and came primarily from the under 25 age group. Males were more likely than females to *never* tell anyone, and much less likely to tell as a child. In a clear majority of cases the writers referred to sexual abuse (80%) and in 23% of cases the sexual abuse was cited along with other forms, most commonly physical and 'mental abuse.' Physical abuse was referred to in 33% of the letters, though only in 3% as a single category; 22% wrote about emotional abuse and 2% referred to neglect. Sexual abuse was the only form of abuse specified in 52% of the letters. However, it should be noted that emotional abuse was seen as accompanying other forms of abuse. Where that was the case it was often the emotional abuse that was considered most damaging with one survivor commenting: 'Although the sexual abuse was horrific the emotional abuse was far worse and had more of a lasting effect on my life.'

The implications for general practitioners and primary health care teams are that many of the adult survivors who present to them have particularly experienced sexual abuse which has usually been accompanied by emotional abuse. However, the consequences and lasting effects of neglect and physical abuse are less well researched and documented. One adult told the National Commission 'I suffered years of physical and mental abuse at the hands of my mother. The hitting stopped when I was sixteen years old but the mental abuse carried on until I was twenty'.

Wattam and Woodward looked at the experiences of child abuse victims and this showed that many may seek help in adulthood

> I would be very grateful if you would please supply me with some contact numbers or addresses to assist me with a problem that has been with me for over 28 years. I am 41 years old, and at the age of 13–16 years I was abused by my father . . . I have never been able to talk to anyone about this matter but I now feel that the time has come.

However, responses to telling in adulthood can be very mixed

> Then I made a major mistake, I told a mate at work about some of the things that had happened to me but not enough that he should call me a poof every time he sees me! I had to leave that job because of the pressure, and believe me it was a blessed relief to go.

Wattam and Woodward coded whether the type of responses that the individual received when he or she told someone about the child abuse that they had suffered was positive or negative. For both children who told about the abuse as children and adults who told as adults, the responses were much more likely to be negative or neutral than positive. Only about one third of adults felt they were supported. The response that is received is an influence on what steps the survivor will take next.

> One particular night I was so upset and my boyfriend persuaded me to tell my mum. I was then 18 years old and finally plucked up the courage to do this. I honestly wish I hadn't. After I told her she just turned round and said 'Well if he comes to the door tell him to go away.' . . . I was upset by the fact she said there was nothing she could do. She didn't even give me a hug.

People do not tell others about their abuse for a number of reasons. When they are children they may not realize that the abuse was wrong. Sadly, they may even consider it to be a feature of normal everyday life.

> When I was about five I was being sexually abused by my two brothers who were about 18 years old.

> All my life has been filled with abuse of one kind or another, so for many years although I knew it was wrong, I thought it was normal and that everyone had secrets. At the time I never knew that it was wrong but I was forced not to tell anyone so I didn't.

As people grow older they may be reluctant to tell someone about their abuse for fear of being considered 'ignorant' or 'silly' – how could they possibly not know that what was happening to them was wrong or think it normal? How could they possibly put up with abuse and not tell anyone? This factor will affect adults' willingness to talk about their childhood experiences. Many abused children also relate how they will not tell about the abuse because they are very afraid of the abuser, they are being blackmailed, or they fear the consequences of telling – for example, that their family will get broken up. These pressures can continue to exert a powerful influence on the individual into adulthood. The individuals might also have very ambivalent feelings towards the abuser – for while they may hate the abuse, in the rest of their lives they may feel so lonely, unloved, and unwanted that they welcome the attention.

Another key factor is the strong feeling of *blame* – the child or the adult survivor may feel that he or she is in some way to blame or responsible for the abuse or that they 'asked for it'. Abusers will encourage this feeling and say that it was the child's fault, and these feelings can be perpetuated into adulthood. The fear of not being believed by family, friends and professionals also exerts a powerful influence on the child or adult survivor not to tell. If someone plucks up the courage to tell someone about their abusive experience and they are not believed by the person they hitherto trusted, they will be less willing to tell someone else. They may not want to expose their vulnerability again.

Primary health care teams may thus encounter adults who have never told anyone, either as children or in adulthood, about the child abuse that they have suffered. But even adults whose abusive experiences were identified while they were children may experience difficulties in adulthood which result from abuse. The consequences of the abuse may never have been addressed. This may be because until recently – and, indeed often still today – responses to child abuse have concentrated on the investigation of the incident. Very little priority has been given to the provision of treatment or therapeutic support. Moreover, survivors told the Commission that when help and support was offered, it was often very short term and inflexible. It seemed that there was no choice – they either had to accept the provision that was proposed or receive no help. It was inflexible because the treatment was being offered only *then* and if it was rejected it would not be offered again. Survivors wanted the option of returning to treatment at a later stage but this was rarely possible, despite the fact that their circumstances and needs changed and that past events would resurface, often triggered by particular events. Survivors also reported that they sometimes felt that the professional supporting them did not really understand either their problem or needs and that the response, as a result, was inappropriate.

Effects of child abuse in adult life

It is now recognized that child abuse can have both short and long term effects that can last into adult life. Some children who have been abused are able to recover from the experience. They are fortunate and their recovery may relate to the nature of the abuse and the extent to which they are provided support at the time. We know that others can experience pain and distress as adults. Wattam and Woodward (1996) suggest that some individuals who did not experience direct effects of abuse as children start to feel the consequences as adults

> I didn't know any different. I didn't know a life of a happy child. I didn't know a life with
> a loving mother and so, I didn't miss it . . . It's only afterwards – when you get older and

the suffering you had starts eating you up inside – because it's stopped – because you no longer have to put shutters up, because you start to realize that your attitudes towards life and people is different from others. It's only then that you really start to become 'messed up' and pay for what you went through all those years ago.

506 survivors who wrote to the National Commission identified the personal experiences of the abuse that they encountered in adulthood. Wattam and Woodward (1996) classified these effects in Table 10.1.

The words of the survivors graphically describe their feelings

Over the last four to five years, I have taken a lot of overdoses, mainly because I feel so unclean. I feel I won't be clean till the day I die.

There is one thing I cannot forget is when I was abused, I was told that I was the double of my mother. Now if anyone says to me how much my mother and I look alike all the memories come back – how can I forget when it's always there . . . The torment never leaves me.

The effect [the abuse] has on me is that as I am naturally shy I tend to retreat into my shell even more deeply and I have difficulty in trusting people, which means I tend to put up a barrier between them and myself.

Many of the survivors spoke about the effects of the abuse on their relationship with family members, present spouses and partners, and others. Some reported that relationships with their family of origin remain difficult or damaged. Their response may be to cut themselves off from their families, particularly blaming their mothers for what happened to them. This can mean that they cut themselves off from support.

Table 10.1 Personal effects in adulthood (n = 506)

Effect	Percentage
Mental health effects (including suicide attempts, depression, breakdown and clinical conditions)	31
Still think about the abuse (including nightmares and flashbacks)	20
General problems (including mood swings and emotional 'damage')	13
Social problems (including alienation, no trust in others)	11
Anxiety (including fear and panic)	7
Eating disorder	7
Addiction (drugs and/or alcohol)	4
Health	4
Other (including positive or no effect, sexual identity)	2

Wattam and Woodward 1996.

Relationships with spouses and partners can also be strained and the abuse is felt to be the cause of this.

Wattam and Woodward (1996) suggest that of those commenting on their relations with spouses and partners, 18% pointed to sexual relationship problems:

> I just feel as if I am not capable to have a relationship or to even do things in a relationship that should be done. Sometimes when we make love I don't think it is right. I think it is dirty for the things he wants me to do to him.

The abuse can also affect other social relationships in adulthood, particularly with men, and in social and work life. 'I find now that I am not comfortable in a man's company. My own marriage broke up and I was never able to have any children either. I blame my father for all that.'

The impact on their own children

Of the thousand people who wrote to the Commission, 32% provided information on how they felt the abuse had affected relationships with their own children. Some of the survivors suggested that their own childhood experiences had enhanced their ability to love, care for, and protect their own children – many were determined that their own children should not have the sort of childhood that they had been forced to endure. Some writers were keen to reject the notion that children who are abused may become adult abusers. This was found to be deeply offensive. However, Wattam and Woodward (1996) point out that:

> The wide range of effects which were reported may have secondary consequences for children – for example, living with a mother who is chronically depressed – many of which must have been extremely difficult for respondents to deal with. At the extreme end this would include the mother who attempted to kill both herself and her children in a desperate plea for help, the mothers who lost their children as a consequence of their mental state and those who were made infertile by the abuse experience. There were also stories from mothers who lost time with their children through hospitalization or depression or who felt they had not been good parents because they were afraid to show affection... A small minority of writers reported serious consequences which included their own children being abused by the person who had abused them.
>
> Wattam and Woodward (1996 pp. 99–100)

Ann Buchanan has considered a number of studies and concludes that there is a very wide variation in rates of intergenerational abuse. She notes that:

> Egeland, Kaufman and Zigler, and Oliver all conclude that intergenerational transmission is far from inevitable... When methodological considerations are taken into account, they conclude it is probable that between 30 and 40% of abused children go on to abuse their children.
>
> Buchanan (1996)

She goes on to quote Kaufman and Zigler, who contend that

> It is time to focus... on the understanding the mechanisms of abuse... Undoubtedly a history of abuse is a considerable risk factor... but the pathway to abusive parenting is

far from inevitable and involves many complex interactions between genetic and environmental factors.

Adult survivors' experiences of services

Those adult survivors giving evidence to the National Commission commented on the help that they had received as adults and the effectiveness of the services they received. This broke down into informal and formal sources of help. Informal help included support from partners, family, and friends and self-help strategies. It is important to see families as a help resource and to offer them support, particularly partners or spouses.

The formal help included counselling, mental health services, medical health services, social work, and voluntary sector services, including survivors' groups. Counselling represented the largest category of help, although it was not always clear who was the provider of this service. Wattam and Woodward (1996) point out that almost half of those using counselling services found they were of most help and that some two-thirds of those attending survivors groups and voluntary organizations (Rape Crisis, Samaritans, Relate, NSPCC) also found these most helpful. However, they add:

> Where the form of help came from professional sources such as health, psychiatric and social services these were the least likely to be viewed as the main or best source of help. Just over a quarter found psychiatric and social services most helpful and only 10 per cent found medical services were the best source of help. GPs in particular were criticized although there were good examples of good practice where GPs referred on to other more appropriate sources of support.
>
> Wattam and Woodward (1996 p. 105)

Gorman undertook a piece of work for the National Commission of Inquiry into the Prevention of Child Abuse which sought to estimate the financial costs of individual cases of child abuse. He analysed nine cases and looked at the costs in relation to the individual's needs as a child and also as an adult (Gorman 1996). The costs break down into two areas: direct costs and indirect costs.

Direct costs include such items as:

- Child protection investigations
- Case conferences
- Fostering
- Individual treatment.

Indirect costs include:

- Delinquency
- Truancy
- Criminal activity and imprisonment
- Mental health services responding to mental distress
- Costs of medication

- GP consultations
- Time out of employment
- Marriage guidance counselling.

Gorman's work illustrated that the costs of responding to the needs of adults abused as children can be significant. The psychological and physical damage caused by abuse can contribute to difficulties in finding and retaining unemployment. We know that adults abused as children are over-represented in the populations of both prisons and psychiatric hospitals. Inpatient psychiatric care and prison both cost on average £20–40,000 per person per year. It would make economic sense to provide help and support to adults who were abused as children. For a comparatively small amount of money, adults abused as children could be more effectively supported and the costs on other services reduced. It is deeply regrettable that, with some notable exceptions, very little consideration is being given by politicians, policy makers, or practitioners to how the needs of adults abused as children can be met.

False memory syndrome

In the late 1980s and 1990s the accuracy of some accounts by adults of their childhood experiences were questioned. It was suggested that they had 'false memories' which had been generated by some forms of therapy. The NSPCC has argued that it is a cause for concern that the justified criticisms of memory recovery therapy have been generalized to cover therapy as a whole, so deterring some adults who were abused as children from seeking help. There is also a risk that public scepticism about the existence of abuse and concern about false allegations will be increased by the controversy over the issue, so that children currently being abused and those who may be at risk in the future will be increasingly disregarded.

Many of the adults who have provided details about the abuse they experienced in childhood – including those quoted by the National Commission and cited in this chapter – have not undergone therapy of any sort and so cannot have been subjected to recovered memories. Dale reports on a ten day international symposium attended by researchers and practitioners to address these issues (Dale 1999). The meeting reached agreement on a number of key principles, including the following:

1 Child abuse is a widespread phenomenon which causes significant harm.

2 Most adults who were abused as children have always been aware of all, or the most salient parts, of their abuse experiences.

3 A small proportion of adults abused as children report that there were periods in their lives when they had no conscious knowledge of their abuse – only to become aware of this in later life. Explanations for such periods of non-awareness remain uncertain and disputed.

4 False beliefs/memories/allegations of childhood abuse do occur. For example, inaccurate abuse 'memories' can be the product of delusional psychiatric states influenced by the topical high public profile of abuse. Another contributory factor is bad therapy with highly suggestible and vulnerable clients (Dale 1999 p. 200).

Most practitioners would now agree that the accounts of abuse provided by both children and adults commenting on what happened to them in childhood should be treated seriously and an effective response provided.

The effectiveness of services to support adult survivors

A recurring theme in the testimonies of adults who were abused as children is that there is a great lack of services and therapy available to them. This is incontrovertible, and it led the National Commission of Inquiry into the Prevention of Child Abuse to conclude that there was an absolute shortage of treatment services and to recommend 'The establishment of a national body for survivors, to act as an information exchange, provide support to member groups and individuals, perhaps through a 24 hour helpline, and undertake development work' (National Commission of Inquiry into the Prevention of Child Abuse 1996 Volume 1, p. 72).

While the accounts of many adults who were abused as children point to the short-comings of the services that they have received, this often because the services provided were considered inappropriate. Many survivors complained of over-reliance on medication. The challenge to professionals is to ensure that services offered are sensitive to the needs of the individual. This is possible and there are many practitioners and survivors' groups that are responding in an appropriate way. We need many more such services.

Peter Dale has looked at the experiences of counselling and psychotherapy by adults who were abused as children. His research involved in-depth interviews with fifty three participants who were clients who had received therapy relating to the consequences of child abuse; therapists who provide such therapy; or therapists who were themselves abused as children. The major conclusion from Dale's research 'is that therapy has the potential to facilitate considerable positive changes for adults who were abused as children – and also that poor therapy can cause significant harm.' He asked the respondents about the quality of their lives before receiving therapy and heard how

> Everyday experiences continually reinforced low self-esteem and chronic lack of self worth. Some had been fixed on self-destructive pathways which included combinations of great loneliness; chronic suicidal preoccupations and attempts; repeated self harming; a range of addictions; repetitive destructive relationships; as well as aggression and abuse of others, including their own children.
>
> Dale (1999 p. 63)

Dale found that 40% of his sample had wholly positive experiences of therapy, leading him to suggest that this 'pays tribute to the skills, thoughtfulness and sensitivity of many members of the therapeutic community and the potential for therapy to be helpful and efficacious' (Dale 1999 p. 195) He writes that the respondents comments on the benefits of their therapy:

> Ranged from general remarks such as literally being life-saving to details of very specific outcomes such as reduction in panic attacks, being able to control emotions, not being depressed, increased self esteem and learning how to communicate in a clear way.
>
> Dale (1999 p. 63)

However, it is a cause for concern that Dale found that some clients experiences were ineffective, unhelpful, and 'sometimes profoundly damaging'. This indicates a need for general practitioners and their primary health care teams to ensure that the treatment received by their patients is effective in meeting the individual's needs, and not damaging.

The Breakfree experience

General practitioners and primary health care teams can make a significant contribution to meeting the needs of adults who were abused as children. There are examples of individual practitioners working on a one-to-one basis with adults and being involved in setting up and supporting survivors' groups. Some individual adults abused as children report that the services they received have been helpful, but examples of specialist services that have been evaluated are rare. Moreover, very few such services have been established. A pilot service, Breakfree, in Lincoln, was evaluated and showed positive outcomes in the short term (Smith *et al.* 1995). Breakfree was set up in the mid-1990s offering care, therapy, and support specifically to adults with a history of child abuse. An evaluation of 116 users over the period of a year was conducted by the project, and staff from Queens Medical School Nottingham, and the Department of Psychiatry, Southern General Hospital, Glasgow.

The adults taking part in the evaluation of Breakfree had been sexually abused as children and had previously received help from health services and other agencies, without much apparent effect. They were frequent users of the health services and their psychological scores indicated that they were very distressed. The research found that Breakfree clients improved significantly in their psychological scores, social activities and distress scale, general health, and delusions, symptoms and states inventory. Smith and his colleagues write that the improvements were:

> Most pronounced for those who had completed therapy by the end of the study. Whereas 82/88 clients had a score for the general health questionnaire that indicated clinical distress at the start, only 25/58 did so at the end of the study (only 17/35 among those who had finished therapy).
>
> Smith *et al.* (1995)

Breakfree offered a comprehensive user-defined package of care within a multi-agency setting. The services provided included:

+ Individual therapy focusing on the abuse with a nominated support worker. The length of session was negotiated with the support worker and was usually 30 to 120 minutes once or twice a week.
+ Day time 'drop in' facility and telephone contact.
+ Out-of-house paging service.
+ Befriending service. This was limited. The support worker offered support, comfort and care to clients who had no support network.
+ A limited 'time out' facility. A client could stay in a safe environment for one or two nights.
+ Support for family and close friends at the client's request.

Smith and colleagues have described the service, as it then operated.

> Breakfree ... is housed in a separate building in a primary care complex. The team consists of Breakfree's originator; a medical director who is also a local general practitioner; and several support workers, all of whom received training in humanistic counselling, specialist training focusing on the abuse itself, and training in allied subjects, such as child protection and offenders' behaviour. The support workers had already expressed an interest in working with adults who had experienced sexual abuse as children, and most came from agencies where they encountered such adults ... All the key local agencies – social services, the area child protection committee, the probation service, the police, the victim support scheme and the National Society for the Prevention of Cruelty to Children – participated in setting up the service and have continued to influence it through an advisory committee.

The authors concluded that the service was effective in the short term and that if the benefits were sustained they would yield a net save in costs to the health service. They added that:

> The traditional health services have clearly failed adults who have experienced sexual abuse as children; these adults continue to show their distress through increased use of health services. All doctors and nurses should become sensitive to the possibility of previous sexual abuse being an underlying problem for patients, and specialist services such as Breakfree should exist to treat these patients.
>
> Smith *et al.* (1995)

Unfortunately, not long after the completion of its pilot, the Breakfree service was discontinued.

The response of GPs and primary health care teams to adults who were abused as children

Adults who were abused as children can face significant health problems that they may raise overtly or covertly with health professionals. These professionals need to know how to respond. The experience of many adults who were abused as children is that the responses are often unsympathetic and unhelpful. Many of the principles that apply to work with abused children can be applied to work with adult survivors. Steps which general practitioners, midwives, health visitors and other primary health care workers can take include the following

+ *Listen carefully and respectfully to what the patients tell you.* This may take time and listening should not be rushed. Adults who were abused as children often report that they are not listened to and feel they are not believed. They recount how it often takes enormous courage and they feel very nervous about telling someone – either a professional or a friend. They feel very let down and rejected when what they say is dismissed. They also report that previous hostile and negative reactions from professionals discourage them from seeking help again. As with children and child abuse, professionals should take very seriously what adults are saying about their childhood experiences. Professionals need to understand that many cases of child abuse are not reported.

◆ *Professionals and the services they provide need to be accessible and non stigmatizing.* Formal services are often criticized by potential users for being unwelcoming, and this makes the task of telling or seeking help more difficult.

◆ Similarly, *professionals should provide information on their services.* Not having information stops people from seeking help. If they do not know what services are provided they cannot know how to access them. Members of the primary health care team can display posters and provide leaflets and information sheets which can be made available at their premises or in outreach settings such as ante natal classes.

◆ *Learn about the consequences of child abuse in adulthood* and understand that some of the patients' symptoms or behaviour may be the result of abuse in childhood. Also recognize that emotional distress and physical ill-health may be triggered by certain events such as becoming pregnant, the onset of adolescence, problems with adult relationships, concerns about parenting skills, and even high profile abuse cases hitting the headlines. The patients' needs may also change over time, with stressful periods being caused by these events.

◆ There is thus a need for *professionals to provide a flexible range of services or make referrals to other professionals and agencies.* Adults abused as children often complain of treatments over-relying on medication. General practitioners and their colleagues need to be aware of the range of possible responses and treatments that may be available locally. For some adults, 'informal' sources of help, including survivors' groups, may be beneficial. However, these groups can be very transient or short lived so it is important that the primary health care team keeps up to date on the availability of such services. Practitioners also need to be aware that these groups, like many counselling services, are not regulated and that they should be used carefully. Local voluntary services that may be of benefit to adults who were abused as children include Relate, MIND groups, and Samaritans. The NSPCC Child Protection Helpline is a 24-hour freephone service that can provide advice on access to services (Telephone 0808 800 5000).

◆ *GPs, midwives, health visitors and other primary health care workers need to act within their competence.* They need to know when to refer on to other specialist services that might include community psychiatric nursing, psychiatric services, counselling or therapy, and social work. Training should address this issue.

◆ *Practitioners need to be aware of sources of practical help that might benefit their patients who were abused as children.* As a result of the effects of childhood abuse, these patients may face problems such as unemployment, poverty, poor housing, and loneliness. Health professionals need to know which local agencies can help with these difficulties. Citizens advice bureaux can be a useful starting point.

◆ *Adults who were abused as children may benefit from help with parenting and the care of their children.* Some survivors have reported that their experiences of child abuse have given them the strength and determination to be 'good' parents and to ensure that their children do not endure the experiences that they did. However, some adults report difficulties in looking after their own children and feel that their confidence has been undermined. GPs, midwives, and health visitors can help support these parents and, where appropriate, refer them to other statutory and voluntary sources of help such as family centres and support groups, Homestart, Newpin, NSPCC, NCH Action for Children and Children's Society family support projects.

- *Outreach work should be undertaken to provide services to that socially excluded group of young people and adults who have no fixed address and are not registered with a doctor.* Primary health care teams, health authorities, and trusts need to work together to meet the needs of this group of patients, a significant proportion of whom will have experienced abuse.

- *The needs of carers and other family members should be considered by the primary health care team.* The effects of child abuse on adults can place considerable strain on the adult's relationships with their partners and families. In some cases partners will have a caring role and need support.

- *Consideration should be given to child protection concerns.* The patient who was abused as a child may be seeking help because she or he has concerns that the abuser is still a risk, perhaps to the patient's own children. In some cases the adult who was abused in childhood may be a risk to his or her own children. In these cases the health professional will need to follow inter-agency procedures as have been described elsewhere in this book.

- *GPs and health visitors could have a role as advocates for adults who were abused as children.* Members of primary health care teams are well placed to understand the needs of this group and can help represent them and advocate on their behalf. Health workers are the professional group most likely to have contact with survivors and there are examples of practitioners who have been instrumental in setting up survivors' groups and other services.

This chapter has sought to illustrate the effects of abuse faced by adults who harmed and neglected as children. Their needs invariably go unrecognized. At present adult survivors face a dearth of services – both statutory and voluntary – and many are forced to suffer significant levels of physical and mental distress in silence. This suffering can be alleviated or eliminated and primary health care workers could play a key role in providing appropriate responses. With improved understanding of child abuse, it is a small step for general practitioners and their primary health care colleagues to meet the needs of adults who were abused as children. Adults who were abused as children do not have to be forgotten patients, and health professionals should have a responsibility to respond.

Sources of help and support

British Association for Counselling and Psychotherapy
1 Regent Place
Rugby
Warwickshire CV21 2PJ
Telephone 01788 550899 E-mail bac@bac.co.uk

NAPAC (National Association for People Abused in Childhood)
c/o BSS, Union House
65–69 Shepherds Bush Green
London W12 8UA

NSPCC Child Protection Helpline
Telephone 0808 800 5000
Textphone 0800 056 0566
E-mail help@nspcc.org.uk

Relate (National Marriage Guidance)
Herbert Gray College
Little Church Street
Rugby
Warwickshire CV21 3AP
Telephone 01788 573241
E-mail enquiries@national.relate.org.uk

Samaritans
10 The Grove
Slough SL1 1QP
Helpline 08457 909090
E-mail jo@samaritans.org

References

The quotes in this chapter from adults who were abused as children are drawn from the letters received by the National Commission of Inquiry into the Prevention of Child Abuse and published in *Childhood Matters* Volume 2.

Buchanan A (1996) *Cycles of Child Maltreatment: Facts, Fallacies, and Intervention.* Chichester: John Wiley and Sons.

Cawson P, Wattam C, Brooker S and Kelly G (2000) *Child Maltreatment in the United Kingdom: A Study of the Prevalence of Child Abuse and Neglect.* London: NSPCC.

Dale P (1999) *Adults Abused as Children: Experiences of Counselling and Psychotherapy.* London: Sage Publications.

Gorman P (1996) The cost of child abuse: some case histories, in National Commission of Inquiry into the Prevention of Child Abuse *Childhood Matters, Volume 1.* London: The Stationery Office.

National Commission of Inquiry into the Prevention of Child Abuse (1996) *Childhood Matters, Volumes 1 and 2.* London: The Stationery Office.

Pearce L and Smith D (1994) *The Breakfree Pilot Evaluation.* Lincoln: Breakfree.

Smith D, Pearce L, Pringle M and Caplan R (1995) Adults with a history of child sexual abuse: evaluation of a pilot therapy service. *British Medical Journal* 310: 1175–8.

Wattam C and Woodward C (1996) 'And do I abuse my children?...No!', in National Commission of Inquiry into the Prevention of Child Abuse, *Childhood Matters, Volume 2.* London: The Stationery Office.

Chapter 11

Domestic violence and child protection: Issues for the primary care team

Leslie L. Davidson and Margaret A. Lynch

Introduction

All professionals who provide care for children and their families must acknowledge the vulnerability of children living in families where domestic violence is present. If a member of the primary care health team (PCHT) identifies domestic violence within a family, then the adverse impact on child welfare must be actively considered. In particular, the co-occurrence of physical and emotional child abuse with domestic violence must be borne in mind and referral to Social Services may be necessary. Even when children are not as yet suffering demonstrable significant harm, they may well meet the criteria for *Children in Need* as defined in the Children Act of 1989, and subsequently benefit from an assessment following the new Framework for Assessment of Children and their Families (Department of Health 2000a). Conversely, in situations where child protection is being considered (such as a child protection case conference), domestic violence is often not recognized. Furthermore, when recognized, the implications of domestic conflict upon child welfare are infrequently addressed during the assessment of risk process or following definition of child protection plans (Farmer and Owen 1995).

This chapter will:

♦ briefly review what is known of the coincidence of domestic violence and child abuse;

♦ consider the adverse effect of domestic violence on children;

♦ describe the policies of relevant professional organizations and the Department of Health;

♦ consider supportive approaches within primary care;

♦ suggest solutions to address specific situations.

Definition of domestic violence

The definition of domestic violence currently used by the Home Office and later adopted in the Department of Health in its publication *Domestic Violence: A Resource Manual for Health Care Professionals* (Department of Health 2000b) is as follows:

> Domestic violence shall be understood to mean any violence between current or former partners in an intimate relationship, wherever and whenever the violence occurs. The violence may include physical, sexual, emotional or financial abuse.

This definition is gender neutral. Although males are also possible victims, over-whelmingly it is women who will experience repeated violence and the more serious consequences of domestic violence. The chapter is therefore written in reference to women experiencing violence and uses the female pronoun.

Violence between adult partners occurs in all social classes, all ethnic groups and cultures, all age groups, in disabled people as well as able-bodied. It may involve abuse, accusation and innuendo; deprivation of freedom; physical or sexual assault; or attacks with deadly weapons.

Background – domestic violence and child abuse

Children's experience of domestic violence in the home

Domestic violence is common and accounts for one quarter of all violent crime in the UK. The recent British Crime Survey (BCS) (Home Office 1999) found that one in four women and one in seven men have been physically assaulted by a current or former partner. Half of those who experienced violence in the past year were living with children under 16, and 29% of these said the children had been aware of what was happening. Not surprisingly this proportion increased to 45% in the families of women who were repeatedly assaulted. It should be remembered that hearing an assault take place can be as distressing for a child as witnessing one.

Experiencing domestic violence results in trauma beyond that of the injuries inflicted. In the BCS, 90% of women reported serious emotional distress as a result of experiencing violence. Over three-quarters of those experiencing chronic violence were very fearful. The emotional difficulties arising for a mother in this situation can impair her ability to care for her children as well as she might wish.

Coincidence of child abuse and domestic violence

The various forms of family violence do not occur in isolation. Violence and abuse may occur in the same family. Children, parents and their partners, and older members may be victims or perpetrators, and may switch roles at different times in the life cycle of the family (Browne and Herbert 1997). When spouse abuse occurs, there is a high possibility that child abuse is also occurring, and vice versa. Edleson (1999) reviewed 35 studies that reported an overlap and concluded that in 30 to 60% of families where either domestic violence or child maltreatment was identified, the other form of violence was also found to be occurring. Walker (1984) in the US found that 53% of men who use violence against their partner also abuse their children. In the

UK Farmer and Owen (1995) identified domestic violence in at least 52% of 44 abusive and neglectful families. It should also be recognized that physical abuse is not always just at the hands of fathers. Straus and Gelles (1990) reported that battered women are more than twice as likely to physically abuse their children. Children are also at risk of injury when they attempt to intervene to protect a parent. A UK study by Glaser and Prior in 1997 found that 28% of 85 children placed on Child Protection Registers for emotional abuse were living in violent households. Few studies have specifically looked at domestic violence and neglect, but the indications are that there is a least a moderate association.

Consideration must be given to both short and long term consequences for the child who lives with domestic violence (Hall and Lynch 1998). The adverse effects appear to depend more upon the intensity and frequency of the violence rather than on their gender or age. The presenting features are varied and may include a tendency to violence, bullying, educational failure and exclusion or dropping out of school. An increased incidence of attention deficit hyperactivity disorder has also been described (Holden and Ritchie 1991; Wolfe *et al.* 1985, 1986). If the mother moves house frequently, or enters a refuge to escape her violent partner, social isolation and loss of friends may add to the child's insecurity.

Current policies and guidelines on domestic violence

There has been a growing interest in domestic violence and health on the part of professional and government bodies over the last five years. As a result, the NHS, the Department of Health and many professional organizations in the Health Care sector have recently issued guidance or policies.

A joint letter about domestic violence from the Director of the Health Services and the Chief Inspector of the Social Services was circulated to all Chief Executives of Health Authorities and of NHS Trusts, Regional Nurse Directors and Directors of Social Services in November 1997. This letter was triggered by a change in civil law under Part IV of the Family Law Act which came into operation in 1996. The joint letter was in the form of helpful guidance for those working within the health and social services, in order to increase knowledge and awareness of domestic violence as a health issue. In addition, the circulation of the joint letter from NHS and Social Service executives underpinned the advice contained in the letter to promote multi-agency work to address domestic violence. The letter defined domestic violence, outlined appropriate responses when domestic violence was identified, and promoted an understanding of the legal context of domestic violence for health professionals and organizations. It specifically targeted primary care, accident and emergency and gynaecology and obstetric services.

As part of the guidance, an appendix was attached giving specific information about how to increase professional's awareness of domestic violence. The letter suggested asking initial questions about overall social and emotional well being (e.g. 'Is everything all right at home?') and following these up with a series of direct questions about potentially abusive scenarios which might be physical and/or emotional in nature. Advice was also provided about making a record of information divulged during such an interview, the autonomy of the patient to refuse this and the legal implications of action taken on behalf of an individual at risk. The NSPCC, the RCN joint working party and a multi-agency project in the London Borough of Camden formally supported the contents of the letter and appendices. This letter was followed up a year later by a reminder and second copy of the letter and by an article in a newsletter sent to all doctors by the Chief Medical Officer of England (Department of Health 1998).

Many professional organizations have published guidelines or recommendations since 1997. These include the following:

- Royal College of General Practitioners (Heath 1998)
- Community Practitioner and Health visitors Association (1999)
- Royal College of Nursing (2000)
- Royal College of Midwives (1997)
- British Medical Association (BMA 1998)
- Royal College of Obstetricians and Gynaecologists (Bewley *et al.* 1997).

While these guidelines do not propose identical recommendations, they all emphasize the prevalence of domestic violence and advocate recognition, assessment and referral within the health services. They focus on multidisciplinary involvement, education and training. These publications aim to raise awareness among their members and to bring institutional change in health care practices.

The main recommendations of the professional organizations centre on improving the identification of women experiencing domestic violence. All cite the need for better information and training about domestic violence and support the need for a non-judgemental and supportive approach. They recommend the development of local policies and guidelines and asking questions about incidents that might be due to domestic violence rather than leaving the victim with the responsibility of bringing up the issue. They all stipulate the need for a safe and private clinical environment. Like the letter to the Chief Executives, they suggest the use of brief initial questions followed up by more detailed enquiry. They cite the need for health professionals to have information on the resources and local initiatives available for women needing referral and include the need for further research to develop appropriate screening tools, strategies to raise awareness and the need for specific training of the professional involved.

Few of the guidelines explore the issue of the overlap between domestic violence and child protection. The RCGP notes it but does not offer suggestions for addressing domestic violence when there are child protection issues, nor assessing the risk to the child when offering assistance to a mother experiencing domestic violence. The CPHVA goes into some detail about the important impact of domestic violence on children, and frames their recommendations in the context of a woman and her children, noting that one reason a woman might not seek help is because of the fear that her children will be put into care (Community Practitioners and Health visitors Association 1999). The RCN notes that child protection procedures must be initiated if the child is in danger, but does not address the wider issues of child welfare (Royal College of Nursing 2000).

The other primary difference between the recommendations centres on when to ask and which women to ask about violence within the context of an intimate relationship. The BMA does not take a position on whether to screen women or not. The RCM recommends asking about violence where the midwife suspects the occurrence of domestic violence. The RCN promotes asking routine questions of all women in many areas of health care, maternity, accident and emergency, mental health, community nursing and health visiting. The RCOG publication recommends asking routine questions about violence of all women who come into contact with the health services through obstetrics, gynaecology, general practice or maternity care.

The focus of the position paper by the Royal College of Midwives (1997) is on the accountability of the midwife alone, though they emphasize the need for a multidisciplinary approach. The RCM paper states minimum standards required by midwives when taking responsibility for women in their care who may be victims or potential victims of violence. This includes documentation and referral and issues around child protection.

The RCOG book *Violence and Women* (Bewley *et al.* 1997), as suggested by its title, goes beyond specialty-specific issues and considers violence and the lives of women. This book adopts a multidisciplinary approach within the health sector, and reviews much of the international research evidence in developing their recommendations.

The British Medical Association report, *Domestic Violence, a Health Care Issue?* (1998) advocates a multi-agency approach and makes recommendations that apply far beyond the health sector. In addition, the BMA broadens the responsibility in the health sector for implementing strategies related to the awareness and management of domestic violence by stating that all Health Authorities should be required to introduce domestic violence into health improvement programmes by consulting and collaboration within a multi-agency setting.

The triennial *Confidential Enquiries into Maternal Deaths 1994–1996* (Department of Health 1998) highlighted violence as a cause of maternal death and made a series of recommendations, broadly based on those of the RCOG, the RCM and the BMA. It supported the following:

- The responsibility of all health professionals to be aware of the importance of domestic violence.

- The development of local strategies and guidelines for the identification and support of women victims including multi-agency working.

- The provision of information about sources of help for victims in clinics.

- That routine questions about violence be included when taking a social history in midwifery, obstetric and gynaecological practice.

- That routine questioning must be accompanied by training for professionals, provision of referral working in collaboration with local groups.

- That interpreters should be provided, if needed, and they should not be a partner, friend or family member.

- That all women are seen on their own at least once during their antenatal care.

These recommendations were accompanied by a Health Service Circular (HSC 1998/1999) issued by the Medical Director of the NHS and the Chief Nursing Officer to all health authorities and trusts and relevant professionals. The circular stated that 'all the recommendations should be implemented as part of local care and audit plans'.

The Department of Health has recently published a resource manual of good practice to help health professionals in a range of settings and for use in the development of local multi-agency protocols (Department of Health 2000b). The resource manual (available free, see resources listed at the end of this chapter) builds on and consolidates the separate guidelines that have been issued by the various Royal Colleges in recent years. It also reiterates the need to link the local Domestic Violence Fora and the Area Child Protection Teams through membership links and through policies.

The recent edition of *Working Together to Safeguard Children*, which was issued in 1999 by the Department of Health, the Home Office and the Department for Education and Employment addresses the co-existence of domestic violence and child abuse. This report includes a thoughtful discussion of the impact of domestic violence on children in the family, even where explicit child abuse or neglect does not occur (*Working Together* 2.21 and 6.38–41), citing the long term impact of witnessing as well as experiencing violence. *Working Together* reviews the inter-agency working necessary to bring the best care and interventions to the family and gives guidance on when to initiate a Social Services assessment of the child or the family (after one serious or several lesser incidents of violence). It is important that the document acknowledges that a range of support services may be needed, as well as assessing the possibility of safeguarding from harm. In particular section 6.40 notes the need to support the non-violent partner.

One of the main conclusions of the 1995 report published by the Department of Health, *Child Protection: Messages from Research*, was that the energies and resources of Social Service departments were overly focussed on investigations and not appropriately targeted on supporting mothers. The report called for a change in the use of resources to give services to mothers earlier, before child protection procedures are brought into play. This policy would be consistent with providing more support and resources for mothers and children where domestic violence is occurring without the need for an explicit child protection investigation. This philosophy is reflected in the recently produced *Assessment Framework for Children in Need and their families* (Department of Health 2000a). This offers the opportunity of a voluntary referral to social services leading to a holistic assessment along three dimensions: the child's developmental needs, parenting capacity and family and environmental factors, with the aim of providing appropriate preventative services to support the family and promote the child's development. The impact of domestic violence and other parental problems including mental illness and substance abuse on children's development is explored in a supporting publication: *Children's Needs – Parenting Capacity* (Cleaver et al. 1999).

The role of primary care

Primary care will have an impact on the effect of domestic violence on the lives of children at several levels. First as members of primary care trusts and commissioning bodies, second as a practice with an ethos and policies, and third on an individual level in primary and secondary prevention and in intervention.

What can Primary Care Trusts (PCTs) do?

The 1998 Crime and Disorder Act requires that local authorities and the police establish local Crime and Disorder Partnerships working together with other relevant agencies, including health. These partnerships are charged to identify the level of domestic violence locally and to include it in their strategy for community safety. There is a need to compile data on the proportion of child protection cases involving domestic violence (Department of Health 2000b). The Home Office has produced a guide for agencies on collecting and managing data that can be accessed at: http://www.homeoffice.gov.uk/violenceagainstwomen/crp.htp.

There is also a requirement for a multi-agency Domestic Violence Forum in every local authority and a recent audit demonstrated that they existed in 93%, but in only 49% was there a representative from the Domestic Violence Forum on the ACPC (Humphreys *et al.* 2000a). The PCG's can be active members of these fora, promoting the liaison between the fora and the ACPC and having a role in developing multi-agency strategies that addresses the whole spectrum of approaches from primary prevention to intervention and rehabilitation. Though domestic violence was mentioned in the Children's Service Plans of 71% of the local authorities in England and Wales, there was provision made in only one fifth of them (Humphreys *et al.* 2000a): the Children's Service Plans are another area where PCGs can have an impact. These groups can commission training for health care professionals, ensure that appropriate information is available to women regarding their rights, and direct them to local resources. The PCGs can consider whether the necessary referral pathways are in place and whether protocols exist.

What can a primary care team do?

A primary care team or practice can be useful in many ways to women and children in families where domestic violence is occurring. Some of these are simple and some are challenging. An essential first step is to provide training to increase the awareness of domestic violence, ensuring that in the training the relationship to child protection is an essential first step. Other key areas include the following:

- Ensuring a supportive and enabling environment in the practice;
- Recognizing that staff themselves may have either been violent or experienced violence at home;
- Ensuring that the practice identifies women experiencing domestic violence;
- Dealing effectively with referrals from other professionals such as midwives;
- Guaranteeing confidentiality to women, except where child protection issues intervene;

- Assessing the risk to the children and determining if the children qualify as children in need or if child protection proceedings should be initiated;
- Considering the safety of the mother and the possible occurrence of domestic violence in any child protection procedures.

Challenges in putting these recommendations into practice

There are serious challenges for primary care teams in putting these recommendations into practice. Few professionals have had adequate training and often feel at a loss when discussing domestic violence with patients. They often feel overwhelmed and impotent in addressing the magnitude of problems which exist (Sugg and Inui 1992; Richardson and Feder 1997). They may be experiencing domestic violence themselves, and this may inhibit or enhance their ability to address this issue with patients. Primary care doctors, unlike most other practitioners, may also care for the person who is being violent and this may be perceived as a conflict for the GP. On the other hand, primary care is an ideal setting for women because it provides confidentiality and the possibility of a trusting relationship linked to continuity of care, characteristics found to be important to women who wish to get help because of domestic violence (Covington et al. 1997).

Women frequently have negative experiences when disclosing domestic violence to health care professionals. One useful study explored the views of abused women about desirable and unwelcome aspects of doctor behaviour and also asked how often the women had encountered each item (Hamberger and Saunders 1998). In a recent review of the North American qualitative literature (Sleutel 1998) women's reports of contacts with health professionals were often negative because of care-givers' tendency to ignore the signs of abuse, or to be unsupportive if they did acknowledge what was happening. If asked, women in the studies covered by Sleutel's review recommended that health professionals ask women about abuse, listen to women and refer them to other sources of help. Women's support for routine screening was high (75%) in one study that asked about it directly (Caralis and Musialowski 1997). This is also supported by a recent survey in Sweden (Stenson et al. 2001).

Henderson (1997) reports the results of a government-sponsored study of domestic violence in Scotland. The views of women experiencing domestic violence were sought by postal questionnaire and by interviews with women contacted through Women's Aid. Similar issues emerged from both sources of information. Women often sought help from GPs and Health visitors; they wanted time to talk and to be taken seriously. They were unhappy with the tendency of some GPs to prescribe medication in response to their visit. Their satisfaction with GPs and Health visitors was primarily linked to the professional's attitude and response, rather than to any practical action taken on the woman's behalf. Some women mentioned that they would like more time to discuss domestic violence during a consultation and would like the caregiver to take the initiative in asking if they had a suspicion that violence was involved.

Training has been shown to have a positive impact on the ability of health professionals to identify and support women. (Thompson RS 1998; McLeer and Anwar et al.

1989) A recent survey of maternity units in England and Wales has found a dearth of training offered to midwives expected to ask women about violence. This same survey found that GPs were the group to whom the maternity units most frequently referred women identified as experiencing violence (Marchant *et al.* 2001). There are some simple steps that can make a difference.

Family violence, alcohol and drug use

Family violence can occur in any family, but where there are difficulties with the use of alcohol or drugs for either the mother or the father, there is a higher than average occurrence of domestic violence and vice versa. Certainly the presence of drug and alcohol problems compounds the difficulties for a family experiencing domestic violence and will increase the challenges in seeking to bring about change or ensure the safety of the mother and children. It is also important to consider domestic violence when assessing a drug or alcohol problem in either mother or father (Berenson *et al.* 1991).

Creating an enabling environment in the practice

In the first instance, a primary care team can create an enabling environment in regard to domestic violence and family violence: this can be accomplished through training, displaying posters and providing information in the office, both in the reception area and in private settings such as the lavatories (with a pen or pencil to copy telephone numbers).

Domestic violence and staff experiences

Because of the prevalence of domestic violence, it is likely that someone in every workplace is herself experiencing violence. Others may be perpetrators. The NHS is one of the largest employers in the UK and can therefore play a role in assisting employees with domestic violence. Very little is written about this. It is mentioned in the CPHVA guidelines (1998) UNISON has published a guide to its members on the importance of making domestic violence a trade union issue (UNISON 1999) and setting out the rationale for workplace policies, taking account of the occurrence of domestic violence.

Ensuring that the surgery environment offers support to those experiencing domestic violence is likely to assist staff as well. The RCN guidance acknowledges the possibility that working with patients experiencing violence may be emotionally difficult and may also raise personal issues as well (Royal College of Nursing 2000). The box at the end of this chapter outlining resources may also be of use to staff individually.

An issue of great importance for primary care staff is their own safety in dealing with issues of domestic violence and child protection. There is also not much written about this, but the Royal College of Nursing has a booklet about the risk of violence to nursing staff which suggests both institutional and individual responses to violence (Royal College of Nursing 1998). This publication focuses more on the violent patient and does not specifically address the risks to staff in working with families experiencing domestic violence. A recent publication, *Social Work, Domestic Violence and Child Protection* (Humphreys 2000b) briefly touches on this issue in regard to social workers, but some of these issues also affect health visitors as well. This document cites employment law, and points towards the need for discussion of difficulties, and for good policy and practice such as doubling up in regard to home visiting in families where domestic violence is known to be occurring.

Assessing the impact on the children

There are a series of specific issues that will come up in clinical practice in reference to the impact of domestic violence on child welfare and possible child protection issues. Whenever domestic violence is identified it is important to consider the welfare of any children living with the woman experiencing violence or the perpetrator (Department of Health 2000b; Mullender 2001).

Domestic violence and children in need

When domestic violence is recognized in a family with children it is important to consider how to approach it, ensuring the welfare and the safety of the children. If the family has come to the attention of the primary care team because of domestic violence issues and not initially because of concerns about child protection, it is still important to consider the following possibilities and make an assessment.

- The child witnesses domestic violence, but no other child protection issue exists;
- Emotional impact on the mother may have an adverse impact on the child;
- The impact of domestic violence in a family may lead to child neglect;
- The child also may be involved in violence, either as a bystander or directly by intervening to protect the mother;
- The child may also be a target of violence.

In making such an assessment, the local ACPC and the designated doctor and nurse may be of assistance. If the assessment finds that there are not direct child protection issues, the children are still likely to qualify as children in need and therefore they and their family require support and assistance. The most recent findings in the Department of Health book *Child Protection: Messages from Research* (1995) was that many families were in need of support and of services and did not receive them. Children of mothers experiencing domestic violence clearly fall into this group, even where there are no direct child protection concerns. *The Framework for the Assessment of Children in Need and their Families* recently published by the Department of Health offers guidance in this area (Department of Health 2000a).

Child protection procedures and the possibility of domestic violence

When the health professional becomes concerned about the presence of child abuse, it is important to consider the safety of other family members: siblings and the mother.

There are many ways in which a health professional becomes aware of domestic violence. The simplest approach is to ask women if they have experienced it. Most research into the views of women has found that women experiencing domestic violence wish and indeed expect the health services to address it with support and referral. Both women who have experienced violence in relationships and those who have not do not mind being asked about violence (Grunfeld *et al.* 1994; Stenson *et al.* 2001; Rodriguez 1996). The RCGP document contains helpful advice on identifying domestic violence as a problem, provides useful questions to ask and advice on confidentiality and documentation. This is available free at www.rcgp.org.uk/rcgp/ corporate/position/dom_violence/index.asp. There are also good examples of how to approach the issue and questions which can be employed in the training packs mentioned below in the box on resources and in the Department of Health resource manual. These also include approaches to recording, risk assessment and information sharing.

Recognizing domestic violence in women

Women disclose occurrence
Bruising – particularly face and neck
Repeated or multiple poorly explained injuries
Frequent A & E visits
Unexplained increase in health care usage
Decrease in preventive care uptake
Repeated failure to attend appointments

When child protection procedures are necessary – approaching issues of domestic violence

In a situation where child abuse or neglect has been identified, it is important to consider whether the mother is also experiencing violence in the family. A study of case conferences occurring in two local authorities found that in 27% of cases coexisting violence towards the mother was known about at the time of the case conference, while in an additional 25% domestic violence was occurring but had not been discovered, and was not addressed at the time of the case conference (Farmer and Owen 1995).

There are simple questions which have been used in the UK to ask the mother about her experience of violence. If violence is occurring the health professional needs to assess the degree of risk to the mother, to offer support and referral to whatever local resources exist. From the start it is essential to provide a safe setting for the mother where requested in all stages of the assessment enquiries and intervention. Advice for health professionals is contained in *Working Together* section 6.41 and may include giving women information about their rights, referral to local agencies, providing practical assistance to enable escape where appropriate and being able to work separately with parents where necessary.

If another agency identifies a child protection issue and if members of the primary care team know that the mother is experiencing domestic violence, they will need to coordinate with the mother when and how to disclose the existence of domestic violence in the family. The GP may need to request that Social Services make special arrangements for the case conference and all other meetings. It may be necessary to arrange that the mother and father attend separately.

Safety of mother during child protection proceedings

A recognition of the frequent coexistence of domestic violence with child abuse has implications for attendance and representation at case conferences: GPs and health visitors need to review the records of parents as well as children. In the case of known domestic violence in the family, there is a need for prior discussion with the mother in regard to disclosure of domestic violence at the case conference. One possible approach may be disclosure in private rather then in an open meeting (i.e. without the father present). The issues of risk to the mother in child contact transfer after divorce have been recently addressed in a report to the Lord Chancellor.

Resources to assist primary care teams

Resources available to primary care teams include the designated doctor and nurse for child protection. There may be a named coordinator for domestic violence in one of the local trusts. Most areas have an active domestic violence fora and national guidance suggests that all ACPC's have protocols regarding the co-occurrence of domestic violence in their policies and procedures (Humphreys *et al.* 2000a). The box below outlines some of the national organizations which give training, produce posters and materials for women or maintain help lines.

Resources and available sources of information for the primary care team and for women

Women's Aid Federation of England

Tel. 0117 944 4411 (office)
Tel. 08457 023468 (helpline)
http://www.womensaid.org.uk (web site)
email: info@womensaid.org.uk

Refuge

Tel. 020 7395 7700 (office)
Tel. 0870 599 5443 (24-hour national helpline)

Victim support national office

Tel. 02077 359166 (office)
Tel. 02077 3030900 (Victim support line)
http://www.victimsupport.com

Resources and available sources of information *(continued)*

Home office telephone for materials address/number

Home Office, PRC Unit Publications, Clive House, Petty France, London SWIV 9HO.
Tel. 020 7271 8225
Fax 020 7271 8344
http://www.homeoffice.gov.uk/domesticviolence

Domestic violence: breaking the chain

Copies of this poster or the booklet are available from HO Marketing Communications Group
Tel. 020 7273 4145
Fax 020 7273 2568

Department of Health

http://www.doh.gov.uk/domestic.htm

Domestic violence

A resource manual for health care professionals – copies available from Department of Health Publications:
Tel. 0541 555455
Fax 01623 724524
E-mail doh@prologistics.co.uk

Domestic violence data source

http://www.domesticviolencedata.org

Training materials

Making an Impact: Children and Domestic Violence Training Pack. School for Policy Studies, University of Bristol, NSPCC, Barnardo's. Available from NSPCC training: 0116 234 0804. This pack contains a reader and training resource with exercises, handouts and materials.

Domestic violence awareness

Training packs for health professionals. Two trainer packs and a trainee pack. Camden Multi-Agency Domestic Violence Forum. Available from: Equalities Unit, Camden Council, room 303, Town Hall, Judd Street, London WC1H 9JE, Tel. 020 7974 6014.

Acknowledgements

We would like to acknowledge the importance of the assistance of Lynne Roberts and Adebimpe Omoseyin, and of building on the knowledge and ideas of Gill Hague, Gene Feder, Jo Richardson, Yvonne Carter, Emma Williams, Judy Shakespeare, Valerie Brasse and others in preparing the chapter.

References

Berenson AB, Stiglich NJ, Wilkinson GS and Anderson GD (1991) Drug abuse and other risk factors for physical abuse in pregnancy among white non-Hispanic, black and Hispanic women. *Am. J. Obstet. Gynecol* 164: 1491–9.

Bewley S, Friend JR and Mezey GC (eds) (1997) *Violence Against Women*. London: RCOG Press.

British Medical Association (1998) *Domestic Violence: a Health Care Issue?* London: BMA.

Browne K and Herbert M (1997) *Preventing Family Violence*. Chichester: Wiley.

Caralis PV and Musialowski R (1997) Women's experiences with domestic violence and their attitudes and expectations regarding medical care of abuse victims. *South Med J* 90(11): 1075–80.

Cleaver H, Unell I and Aldgate J (1999) *Children's Needs – Parenting Capacity. The Impact of Parental Mental Illness, Problem Alcohol and Drug Use, and Domestic Violence on Children's Development*. London: The Stationery Office.

Community Practitioners and Health visitors Association (1998) *Domestic Violence: the Role of the Community Nurse*. London: CPHVA.

Covington DL, Dalton VK, Diehl SJ, Wright BD and Piner MH (1997) Improving detection of violence among pregnant adolescents: systematic violence assessment. *Journal of Adolescent Health* 21(1): 18–24.

Department of Health (1995) *Child Protection: Messages From Research*. London: DoH.

Department of Health (1998) CMO's Update, Letter to Doctors from the Chief Medical Officer. London.

Department of Health, Welsh Office, Scottish Office Department of Health, Department of Health and Social Services NI (1998) *Why Mothers Die. Report on Confidential Enquiries into Maternal Deaths in the United Kingdom 1994–1996*. London: The Stationery Office.

Department of Health (1999) *Working Together to Safeguard Children: A Guide to Inter-agency Working to Safeguard and Promote the Welfare of Children*. London: The Stationery Office. Also on www.doh.gov.uk/domestic.htm.

Department of Health (2000a). *Framework for the Assessment of Children in Need and their Families*. London: The Stationery Office.

Department of Health (2000b) *Domestic Violence: a Resource Manual for Health Care Professionals*. London: DoH.

Edleson JL (1999) The overlap between child maltreatment and woman battering. *Violence Against Women* 5(2): 134–54.

Farmer E and Owen M (1995) *Child Protection Practice: Private Risks and Public Remedies. Studies in Child Protection*. London: HMSO.

Glaser D and Prior V (1997) Is the term child protection applicable to emotional abuse? *Child Abuse Review* 6: 315–29.

Grunfeld AF, Ritmiller S, Mackay K, Cowan L and Hotch D (1994) Detecting domestic in the emergency department: a nursing triage model. *J Emergency Nursing* 20: 271–4.

Hall D and Lynch MA (1998) Violence begins at home. Domestic strife has lifelong effects on children [editorial]. *BMJ* 316(7144): 1551.

Hamberger LK and Saunders DG (1998) Physician interaction with battered women: the women's perspective. *Arch Fam Med* 7(6): 575–82.

Heath I (1998) *Domestic Violence: the General Practitioner's Role*. London: Royal College of General Practitioners. Also at www.rcgp.org.uk

Henderson S (1997) *Service Provision to Women Experiencing Domestic Violence in Scotland*. Edinburgh: Scottish Office Central Research Unit.

Holden GW and Ritchie KL (1991) Linking extreme marital discord, child rearing and child behavior problems: Evidence from battered women. *Child Development* 62: 311–27.

Home Office (1999) *Domestic Violence: Findings from a new British Crime Survey Self-completion Questionnaire*. London: Home Office Research Studies.

Humphreys C, Hester M, Hague G, Mullender A, Abrahams H and Lowe P (2000a) *From Good Intentions to Good Practice: Mapping Service Working with Families where there is Domestic Violence*. Bristol: The Policy Press.

Humphreys C (2000b) *Social Work, Domestic Violence and Child Protection: Challenging Practice*. Bristol: The Policy Press.

Marchant S, Davidson LL, Garcia J and Parsons JE (2001) Addressing domestic violence through maternity services – policy and practice. *Midwifery*, 2001, 17: 164–70.

McLeer SV and Anwar RA (1989a) A study of battered women presenting in an emergency department. *AJ Public Health* 79: 65–6.

McLeer SV, Anwar RA, Herman S and Maquiling K (1989b) Education is not enough: a systems failure in protecting battered women. *Annals of Emergency Medicine* 18(6): 651–3.

Mullender A (2001) Meeting the needs of children in *What Works in reducing domestic violence: A comprehensive guide for professionals* Commissioned by the Home Office, Julie Taylor-Browne, Whiting and Birch (eds). London, 35–9.

NHS Executive. (1998) Health Service Circular. Confidential Enquiries into Maternal Deaths 1994–96. HSC 1998/211.

Richardson J and Feder G (1997) How can we help? – the role of general practice, in S Bewley, JR Friend, GC Mezey *Violence Against Women*. London: RCOG Press.

Rodriguez MA (1996) Breaking the silence. Battered women's perspectives on medical care. *Arch Fam Med* 5(3): 153–8.

Royal College of Midwives (1997) *Domestic Abuse in Pregnancy* (Position Paper No. 19). London: RCM.

Royal College of Nursing (1998) *Dealing with Violence Against Nursing Staff: An RCN Guide for Nurses and Managers*. London: RCN.

Royal College of Nursing (2000) *Domestic Violence: Guidance for Nurses*. London: RCN.

Sleutel MR (1998) Women's experiences of abuse: a review of qualitative research. *Issues in Mental Health Nursing* 19(6): 525–39.

Stenson K, Saarinen H, Heimer G and Sidenvall B (2001) Women's opinion on being asked about exposure to violence. *Midwifery* 17: 2–10

Strauss MA and Gelles RJ (1990) *Physical Violence in American Families: Risk Factors and Adaptations in 8,145 Families*. New Brunswick, NJ: Transaction Publishers.

Sugg NK and Inui T (1992) Primary care physicians' response to domestic violence. *JAMA* 267(23): 3157–60.

Thompson RS (1998) A training program to improve domestic violence identification and management in primary care: preliminary results. *Violence and Victims* 13(4): 395–410.

UNISON (1999) *Raising the Roof on Domestic Abuse: a UNISON Guide to Campaigning Against Domestic Violence*. London: UNISON Communications Unit.

Walker LE (1984) *The Battered Women*. New York: Springer.

Wolfe DA, Zak L, Wilson S and Jaffe P (1986) Child witnesses to violences between parents: Critical issues in behavioral and social adjustment. *J Abnormal Child Psychol* 14: 95–104.

Wolfe DA, Jaffe P, Wilson SK and Zak L (1985) Children of battered women: The relation of child behavior to family violence and maternal stress. *J Consulting and Clin Psychol* 53: 657–65.

Chapter 12

Legal aspects of child abuse

Fran Clift

Introduction and chapter aims

The purpose of this chapter is to provide guidance for primary health care practitioners on legal aspects of the child protection process. The Children Act 1989 ('the Act') is the relevant statute. However, there are areas where common law still applies, for example, consent to treatment and confidentiality. Sometimes there are no strictly 'legal' provisions and in this case, guidelines from the Department of Health, the Medical Royal Colleges and other professional bodies are of great importance for informing best practice. We will look at:

- The principles embodied in the Act;
- The duties of the statutory agencies including health, and their staff, to protect children;
- The orders which the court may make if the test of significant harm is satisfied;
- Patient confidentiality along with legal and ethical considerations for health professionals ;
- Courts including reports, proceedings and giving evidence.

Lastly we look at the legal and professional consequences for healthcare professionals arising from failure to diagnose and report abuse.

Where important principles have been established by case law rather than statute, the case names are given in the text in brackets with the full legal reference at the end of the chapter.

The Children Act 1989

Framework

- The public and private law relating to children is now embodied in the Act. Its overall objective is to balance the interests of children with the responsibilities of their parents. The Act introduced firm measures available for state intervention when necessary within the context of a unified court system.

- The key elements of the Act are: the paramountcy of the child's welfare, the welfare checklist and the '*no order*' principle.
- Part 1 sets out the key principle that in making decisions about a child's upbringing, the child's welfare shall be its paramount consideration. The Act also defines parental responsibility which is of the utmost importance in consent to treatment.
- Part 2 defines the 'private law' orders which the court can make with respect to children (for example, who they live with and have contact with). These orders are made when parents are in dispute but do not involve outside agencies. Healthcare workers may be asked to prepare reports in these proceedings and/or give evidence.
- Part 3 deals with the duty of the local authority to provide support for children and their families.
- Part 4 explains the circumstances in which care and supervision orders may be made. A court may only make a care or supervision order if it is satisfied that the child is suffering or is likely to suffer significant harm attributable to the care being given or is considered to be beyond parental control.
- Part 5 deals with the protection of children including the making of emergency protection orders, orders for medical examinations and the powers of the police to remove and accommodate children in need of protection. Healthcare workers will often be involved in this process, reporting suspected child abuse, carrying out medical examinations, attending case conferences, preparing reports for the court and giving evidence.

Healthcare professionals may be asked to provide reports for the court and/or be required to attend court to give evidence on any of the above points.

- The remaining parts of the Act set out the duties of local authorities to provide and regulate community, voluntary and registered children's homes, fostering, child minding and daycare arrangements, the powers of the secretary of state and miscellaneous matters including the accommodation of children by health authorities and in residential care, nursing homes or mental nursing homes.

The welfare checklist

- Section 1 of the Act states that when a court determines any question with respect to the upbringing of a child, his welfare shall be the court's paramount consideration.
- 'Welfare' is not defined but a checklist of factors is provided which should be considered by courts when making, varying or discharging care or supervision orders. These factors are:
  - The ascertainable wishes and feelings of the child concerned (considered in the light of his age and understanding).
  - His physical, emotional and educational needs.
  - The likely effect on him of any change in his circumstances.
  - His age, sex, background and any characteristics of his which the court considers relevant.

- Any harm which he has suffered or is at risk of suffering.
- The capability of each of his parents, and any other person in relation to whom the court considers the question to be relevant, in meeting his needs.
- The range of powers available to the court under this act in the proceedings in question.

The 'no delay' and non-intervention ('no order') principles

The courts are under a positive duty to ensure that delay in determining a child's future does not occur and that orders are not made unless absolutely necessary. This principle is also reflected in the obligations of local authorities and health bodies to cooperate in the area of child protection to support parents and avoid the intervention of the court if possible.

Parental responsibility

- Section 3 of the Act defines parental responsibility as being all the rights, duties, powers, responsibilities and authority, which by law a parent has in relation to his child and his property.
- Section 2 sets out who has parental responsibility for a child. This will be particularly important where questions of confidentiality and consenting to or refusing medical treatment arise. Those who have it are:
  - Both parents, provided that the father and mother were married to each other between conception and birth or afterwards including where a child is born as a result of a woman being artificially inseminated by sperm not of her husband, provided he consented to it. (cf Section 28, *Human Fertilisation and Embryology Act 1990* i.e. 'HFEA').
  - The mother alone, if the child's parents were not married unless the father has a formal written parental responsibility agreement with the mother or by court order. The government plans to give parental responsibility to unmarried fathers who sign the child's birth certificate jointly with the mother at some time in the future.
  - A guardian appointed by a will or by the court; for example, if the child's parents are dead.
  - A person who has a residence order in respect of the child.
  - Gamete donors whose child has been born as a result of a surrogacy arrangement and who have a parental order made under S.30 HFEA.
  - A local authority where there is a care order or an emergency protection order (though in the case of the latter this is limited).
  - Persons who have an adoption order.

Please note the following:

- Caution should be exercised when dealing with people whose permanent home is not England and Wales, in respect of whom rights may be very different.

+ Except in the case of adoption and parental orders made in favour of gamete donors, the mother or parents never lose parental responsibility for a child, even if another such as a local authority has a care order or the grandmother a residence order. In this case parental responsibility is shared.

Consent to treatment

The law on consent to medical treatment is based on the individual's right to self-determination. Treatment without consent is an assault and may result in civil and criminal proceedings against the health professional. Consent can only be given by a competent adult (In Re C 1994 and Re MB 1997). An adult for this purpose is a person of 16 or over or an under 16-year- old who is Gillick competent (Gillick 1985), in other words has sufficient maturity and intelligence to understand the proposed treatment and its consequences. The determination of Gillick competence will be made by the health professional concerned.

In the case of young children consent must be given by one holder of parental responsibility. Sometimes consent for a medical procedure which doctors believe is in the best interests of a child is refused by the holder of parental responsibility. On the face of it this may raise child protection issues and in any case requires careful handling. If, after all efforts to reach a consensus have failed, a health professional should seek a second professional opinion and advice from management. It may be decided in the case of life saving or other serious treatment to ask the court to make a determination. The court's paramount consideration must be the welfare/best interests of the child and not the views of the parents, though these are very important. Best interests has not been defined as such, but treatment must include a genuinely therapeutic element and the wider welfare, family and social circumstances of the child will also be considered. At this stage the parents must be told to take legal advice and the professional should do the same.

An application will normally be made to the family division of the high court within its inherent jurisdiction for consent to be given for the treatment to go ahead. The court will also be able to grant other orders such as that the child should not be removed from hospital, or not have contact with a person who is impeding treatment.

Responsibility to the child

The Act places specific duties on all social agencies, including healthcare agencies, to cooperate in the interests of vulnerable children

+ Specifically, S.17 makes it the duty of every local authority to safeguard and promote the welfare of children within their area who are in need and, so far as is consistent with that duty, to promote the upbringing of such children by their families.

+ S.27 provides that the local authority (which of all agencies has the primary responsibility for child protection) may request help from Trusts in exercising its function to provide support and services for children in need. The health authority/ trust through its staff has a *duty* to comply.

♦ S.47 places a duty on a health trust to help the local authority with its enquiries where there is reasonable cause to suspect a child is suffering or is likely to suffer significant harm.

♦ The doctor's duty at common law is to treat children in their best interests. There is no specific duty on the doctor under the Act.

♦ The 1999 Department of Health Guidelines *Working Together to Safeguard Children, (Working Together)* (Department of Health 1999) and the accompanying publication *Framework for the Assessment of Children in Need and their Families* (Department of Health 2000) are essential reading for health professionals. They set out how agencies and professionals should work together to promote children's welfare and protect them from abuse and neglect. Although they do not have the force of law the guidelines inform best practice and should be followed. They set out:

• The importance of checking the child protection register if a professional suspects abuse and of contributing to assessments as to whether registration is necessary.

• The need to make it clear on patient records that a child is on the register.

• What to do and who to inform if you suspect abuse.

• The obligation on health authorities and trusts to appoint designated child protection professionals (a paediatrician and a senior nurse) in each area who can provide help to professionals.

• The role of the professional at the child protection conference, on review and in investigations of abuse.

• The role of the Area Child Protection Committee.

• The obligation on employers including GPs to train staff in child protection.

♦ The BMA, GMC UKCC and local Area Child Protection Committees also issue guidance on inter agency cooperation and information sharing.

Public law orders to protect children

Emergency Protection Orders (EPOs)

♦ S.44 of the Act provides that any person, though it will usually be the local authority, occasionally the police and in rare cases a health trust can apply to the court for an EPO and the court may grant it if it is satisfied that:

• There is reasonable cause to believe that the child is likely to suffer significant harm if he is not removed to accommodation provided by or on behalf of the applicant, or he does not remain in the place in which he is then being accommodated.

• In the case of an application made by a local authority, S.47 enquiries are being made but access to the child is being unreasonably refused in circumstances where access is urgent (or enquiries made by others are being frustrated in the same way and there is a likelihood of significant harm).

- Before making the order the court must be convinced that intervention is justified and must apply the welfare test. The order:

  Operates as a direction to produce the child.

  Lasts for 8 days(extendable for a further 7 days).

  Gives limited parental responsibility to the applicant.

  Authorizes or prevents removal of the child from his present accommodation.

- It may also:

  Exclude the perpetrator of harm from the child's home.

  Limit or forbid contact with a parent/s.

  Order a medical examination (which may be refused by a Gillick competent child).

  - No application for the order to be discharged may be made within 72 hours of the order being made.

- S.45(12) enables the court to direct that a health professional accompany the applicant when the order is executed.

- S.46 enables the police to remove a child to suitable accommodation or prevent his removal from hospital or any other place if they have reasonable cause to believe that the child would otherwise be likely to suffer significant harm. Again the court may direct a health professional to accompany the police.

- A recovery order under S.50 enables a child who has run away or is kept from the responsible adult who is supposed to be caring for him to be returned.

- Following the making of an EPO or if a child is in police protection, the local authority is bound to make enquiries (S.47) and decide what further steps should be taken to safeguard and promote the child's welfare. Healthcare professionals have a duty to assist by passing information and attending child protection conferences when required.

- Health professionals are likely to be involved at some or all stages of the EPO and enquiry stages. Medical evidence may be required by the court to enable it to decide whether there is a risk of significant harm, or as to the appropriate order for medical examination. Before a medical examination is carried out it is *essential* to consider who has parental responsibility and whether the child is Gillick competent. In addition health workers have a statutory duty in relation to S.47 enquiries to assist with the passing of information, attending or providing information for child protection conferences and child protection plans.

Child Assessment orders

If, following a S.47 investigation, the local authority or health professional has a real concern that the child may be suffering significant harm but it is not an emergency situation warranting an EPO, the local authority or NSPCC can apply under S.43 for a child assessment order. The order only lasts for seven days and does not give parental responsibility to the local authority, though contact may be prevented if an assessment is to take place in hospital. A medical assessment will usually be required which, again, the Gillick competent child can refuse. It is likely that by this stage there will have been a case conference to which the doctor will have contributed.

Care orders

◆ A care order has the effect of giving the care of a child up to 16 years to the local authority, giving parental responsibility to it and usually means that the child will be removed from home. The court will only make an order if it is convinced that no less drastic remedy such as provision of family services is appropriate. It is made on the following grounds:

- That the child concerned is suffering or is likely to suffer significant harm; and

- That the harm or likelihood of harm is attributable to the care given to the child, or likely to be given to him if the order were not made, not being what it would be reasonable to expect a parent to give to him OR the child is beyond parental control.

◆ The court must consider these grounds within the context of the welfare principle, the check list and the no delay and non-intervention principles.

◆ S.31(9) of the Act defines:

- 'Harm' as ill treatment or the impairment of health or development.

- 'Development' as physical, intellectual, emotional, social or behavioural development.

- 'Health' as physical or mental health.

- 'Ill-treatment' as including sexual abuse and forms of ill-treatment which are not physical.

◆ Significant harm is the threshold which justifies the state's intervention in private and family life, in the best interests of children. There are no absolute criteria on which to determine significant harm but they include the degree and extent of physical harm, the duration and frequency of abuse and neglect and the extent of premeditation, the degree of threat and coercion, and sadism and bizarre or unusual elements in child sexual abuse. Although a single event may meet the criteria, more often it will be a series of events constituting long standing neglect or abuse. See *Working Together* 2.16–17.

◆ The court may need assistance through reports and/or oral evidence from health-care professionals as to whether in their opinion the harm to the child is significant, what standard of care and development would be the norm in a child with similar attributes, as provided by reasonable parents, and whether the harm is attributable to the parents.

Supervision orders

◆ These can be made in respect of a child up to the age of 16 and places the child under the supervision of the local authority or probation officer. Its usual duration is one year. The supervisor must advise, assist and befriend the supervised child S.35(1)(a). The grounds for making it are the same as for a care order, though usually the child will stay at home. The child may be required to participate in certain activities, present himself to the supervisor at certain times and submit to medical or psychiatric examinations. If the examination is to take place in hospital or in the case of a psychiatric examination, a hospital or mental nursing home at which the child is to attend as a residential patient, the court must approve it. It will only do so on the evidence of a doctor that the child may be suffering from a physical or mental condition that requires and may be susceptible to medical treatment, and a period of residence is necessary if the examination is to be carried out properly. If a Gillick competent child refuses the court will not order it.

◆ Similar provisions exist in Schedule 3 of the Act in relation to psychiatric and medical treatment. Here again, the healthcare professional may be asked to carry out examinations, treat the child, write reports, and give evidence or guidance to the court as to what specific examinations and assessments would be appropriate.

Guardians at litem

Guardians work under the auspices of the Children and Family Court Advisory and Support Service (CAFCASS). They represent children's interests in nearly all public law cases. By profession, they are court welfare officers, social workers, or former case workers from the Official Solicitors' office and are appointed by the Court.

They advise the child, arrange for a solicitor to represent the child, investigate and write reports for the court. They will advise a court making an order for medical examination whether the child is Gillick competent, speak to health professionals involved in the child's care and examine social work but not health records unless they form part of the social work records.

Confidentiality and access to records

Requests for access

Requests for access to a child's records may be made by a person with parental responsibility unless:

◆ The information has been given by or the examination carried out on a Gillick competent child in the expectation that it will not be disclosed; or

◆ The appropriate health professional considers that access will cause *serious harm* to the physical or mental health or condition of the child (S.7 Data Protection Act 1998).

Sharing information with other agencies

◆ A patient is entitled to expect complete confidentiality in relation to information given to a healthcare professional in the course of a consultation because the patient gives the information on that basis (Stephens *v* Avery 1988). Breach of confidentiality by a healthcare professional is extremely serious and may result in disciplinary proceedings by his employer and his professional organization and legal action against the professional and the employer for damages unless it can be justified.

- However the duty of confidence is not absolute. *Working Together* places a clear obligation on health professionals to work together with social services and other agencies to promote children's welfare and protect them from abuse and neglect. It is therefore most unlikely that the passing on of confidential patient information to the proper authorities, when a health professional has good reason to suspect significant harm or the likelihood of it, would be viewed as an unjustifiable breach of confidence by a court. The DOH *Guidelines on the Protection and Use of Patient Information* (1996) strengthened by the provisions of the Data Protection Act 1998 also justify it when necessary for the welfare of the child. The GMC has also endorsed this. However the professional should take care to record carefully what information was given, to whom and only to give as much as is necessary to protect the child in question. Assurances should be obtained that the information will not be shared with third parties unless specifically agreed.

- Remember that information given to social services may be regarded as forming part of local authority records, and will be available to a guardian writing a report for court proceedings if the information is given unconditionally.

- A patient should always be told what information will be passed on and to whom unless, in the professional's opinion, it would be harmful to the child to do so. If you have to give evidence it is good practice to inform the parents and explain that the judge will ask questions which you will have to answer. The result may be the destruction of the professional–patient relationship, but the duty to act in the child's best interests is paramount.

- The decision to break a confidence is a difficult and anxious one and will always be a matter of judgement. If in doubt as to whether to share information, seek advice from your manager, the designated paediatrician or nurse in the area or from the trust or GP's legal advisers.

Confidentiality and young people

The duty of confidentiality owed to a person under 16 is as great as that owed to any other person. An explicit request by a patient that information given during a consultation should not be passed on to anyone (often a parent) must be respected save in the most exceptional circumstances, for example where a health professional believes that the young person or their siblings are being abused and it is necessary to share the information to protect them. The professional must try to get the cooperation of the patient to pass on the information, with appropriate counselling, if necessary. If this is impossible, he must tell the patient that he will have to pass on the information. This may destroy the therapeutic relationship, and the professional must be careful to record everything and be able to justify his actions to the GMC or relevant professional body if a complaint is made.

The Human Rights Act 1998

The Human Rights Act came into force on 2 October 2000. It incorporates into domestic law the European Convention on Human Rights which the UK government signed in 1951. Its provisions bind 'public authorities' which include NHS trusts, GPs and healthcare workers employed by them and local authorities. Public authorities are bound to respect and promote the Articles of the Convention.

The most important Article for child protection law is Article 8, the right to respect for private and family life, which provides that:

◆ Everyone has the right to respect for his private and family life, his home and his correspondence.

◆ There shall be no interference by a public authority with the exercise of this right except such as is in accordance with the law and is necessary in a democratic society in the interests of national security, public safety or the economic well-being of the country, for the prevention of disorder or crime, for the protection of health or morals, or for the protection of the rights and freedoms of others.

The right is qualified by its second limb, so there are limits to how the patient can exercise it. For example, the right to respect for a patient's private life is qualified by the necessity to protect the health of others. This will justify a breach of confidence to protect an abused child. The right of a parent to enjoy family life is limited by the child's right to be safe which may justify state interference with the parent's right. Essentially, the Convention is about balancing the rights of one person against another, and society and decisions by a health professional must be able to be justified in those terms. The importance of keeping good records and fully noting the reasons for decisions cannot be overstated.

Court reports

Record keeping

The key to writing useful and accurate reports is to keep good records. What follows may be to state the obvious but it is nevertheless crucial. All records should be dated, timed, signed and written clearly in pen. A useful rule to follow is the four Ws, when (it happened), what (happened), witnessed by (who) and why (it happened/you did what you did). It is important to use terms which are clearly understood and not open to misinterpretation. Remember that the writer of the records may not be the person who eventually writes the report. Do not comment on areas outside your professional expertise. Make clear in the notes your sources of information. Include details of the information and explanations given to child and parent patients particularly when there are sensitive confidentiality or consent issues. If a child is on the child protection register that should be clearly stated in the records of all family members. Write records contemporaneously or immediately after a visit or consultation. Old recording is a standard subject for cross examination. As far as health visitors are concerned there should be no discrepancy in the records kept in the family home and those in clinics or health centres, unless there are exceptional circumstances.

Contents

Reports should begin with the writers qualifications and how long they have been treating the child and his family. Look at the court's directions, if any, as to the required content. Whether the terms are specific or non-existent the same rules apply. Stick to the facts from your records and state them in chronological order, avoid ambiguous sentences which can be picked on by lawyers in cross-examination, make clear sources of information and only report conclusions based on your professional opinion within your own speciality, remembering that the report will be read by non-medical people. Finally, all reports should be referred to the appropriate manager or the GP and thence to the designated senior child protection professional in the area if further guidance is needed. In difficult cases legal advice may be required.

When to write a report

+ If a report is ordered by the court then clearly it must be done. To refuse is a contempt of court punishable by fine or imprisonment. If the health professional is unhappy about an order made in their absence, an application should be made to the court and the judge asked to reconsider or modify the order.

+ If the report is requested by the local authority for court proceedings this is probably because there are child protection issues and the healthcare worker is obliged under S.27 of the Act and *Working Together* to produce it. This can be done without a court order but the employer may require one.

+ Requests for reports in private law proceedings, such as a dispute between parents about residence or contact, usually come from one party's solicitor and should be treated with caution. There may be no child protection issues and the professional's duty of confidence to the parent who has not requested the report will not easily be overcome. In addition the professional may have to continue to work with the whole family once the proceedings are over. It is not easy to convince someone that you are not biased in favour of the person 'for whom' you wrote the report.

+ Unless all parties to the proceedings agree after discussion with them of the contents of the report (so that the confidentiality has been waived), or the contents of the report are completely uncontroversial, it is better to refuse but to say that if the court orders a report it will be provided.

+ Healthcare professionals may be asked to provide a statement for the police in cases where a child has died from abuse or neglect, or where the child has sustained injuries and an adult is being prosecuted for a criminal offence. Some trusts and defence organizations prefer to have a lawyer present when the statement is taken. Read the statement carefully before signing. Changing it later may be refused.

+ If a report is provided following a court order a breach of confidence in the report or in court is justified, provided the general rules are observed (see Section E1–3).

Court

Court structure

Proceedings involving the protection of children can be heard by magistrates' family proceedings court, by designated trial centre county courts or by the family division of the high court. Most public law cases are heard in the magistrates' family proceedings court. Applications involving children in divorce proceedings are heard in the county court. Cases can be transferred from the magistrates to the county court and the high court. The high court will hear the most serious cases particularly those involving complicated medical issues. Criminal prosecutions against perpetrators of abuse will start in the magistrates court and the serious ones will be committed for trial at the crown court.

Appearing in court

◆ When should a healthcare worker agree to attend court to give evidence? If you have written a report by order of a court or at the request of the local authority in family proceedings you should attend court if asked without a witness summons. A breach of confidentiality committed in these circumstances, while giving evidence, can be defended provided the evidence given does not disclose more than is necessary to protect the child. Some employers may require the local authority to obtain a witness summons so consult your manager before committing yourself. In all other circumstances you should ask the person calling you to obtain a witness summons.

Going to court

◆ If you have not given evidence before you may want to take a colleague with you. However, since proceedings (except criminal) are held in private he or she will probably not be allowed to come in to court with you. You should take the original records and any report that you have written, though a bundle containing the report will usually be given to you when you give evidence. If you are unhappy with your report, you can amend it but try to speak to the lawyer who is calling you to warn them.

◆ You will usually go into a witness box to give evidence and be questioned by the lawyer who asked you to come to court first. You will be asked open questions, i.e. those which do not suggest an answer about what happened. If the questions are incomprehensible or are outside your area of expertise, say so. Do not give opinions which you are not qualified to give.

◆ You will then be cross-examined by the other parties' lawyers. These questions will often be closed, suggesting an answer which the lawyer hopes will strengthen their client's case. Do not be caught out by suggestions you do not agree with. Remain alert, stick to the facts and give opinions sparingly in accordance with your expertise. You may then be re-examined by the first lawyer dealing with matters arising from cross-examination. Address all your answers to the judge.

Consequences of wrongly diagnosing, failing to diagnose or to pass on evidence or suspicion of abuse

Negligence

♦ The most likely claim to be brought on behalf of a child is for clinical negligence. Proceedings must be started not later than his twenty-first birthday (Limitation Act 1980). Doctors nurses and other healthcare staff within NHS trusts are covered by the NHS indemnity and their employer will be responsible for providing lawyers and paying any damages awarded. A GP is personally responsible and provided he is properly indemnified his defence organization will provide legal advice and pay the damages. Early reporting of potential claims is essential. Cover is only provided for healthcare professionals acting in their professional capacity in the course of their employment, and in respect of acts or omissions admitted as negligent by the employer or determined as such through the legal process.

♦ For a claim to be successful the child would have to prove:

• That the care provided by the doctor failed to meet the standard of the ordinary skilled doctor exercising and professing to have that particular skill. In the case of a GP, the judge will decide this by hearing expert evidence from (usually) two GPs who also see children who have been abused. The standard is met if it is accepted as proper by a responsible body of medical opinion (Bolam 1957). In other words the doctor's acts must reflect accepted medical practice. However the body of medical opinion must withstand logical analysis by a court i.e. be reasonable and justifiable (Bolitho 1997).

• That the breach of duty has caused a loss. The loss in a case of failure to diagnose child abuse would include physical and psychological damage and in the case of a wrong diagnosis psychological damage. The question for the court is whether, but for the failure to diagnose or the misdiagnosis, the child would have suffered the particular damage alleged? The cause of the loss or damage must be proved on the balance of probabilities, i.e. is it more likely than not?

♦ The damages awarded aim to put the child in the position he would have been in had the negligence not occurred and includes awards for pain and suffering (including psychiatric illness) and past and future financial loss caused by the negligence.

The GMC

A wrong diagnosis of or failure to detect or pass on evidence of child abuse may result in a complaint to the GMC by a parent. Part of the GMC's function is to remove or suspend registration, or put conditions on a doctor's practice when the doctor has been guilty of serious professional misconduct or the doctor's professional performance has been found to be seriously deficient . It is unlikely that a single act of negligent practice would be enough to justify action but a series of acts even if they were honest mistakes may be. The result would be suspension, the imposition of conditions on practice or striking off the register. Clearly, early legal advice is essential.

Inquests

If abuse results in the death of a child then it is likely that an inquest will be held on the ground that it is a violent or unnatural death. If a GP or other healthcare professional has been involved in the care of the child, then he or she will be asked by the coroner's office to provide a statement and then attend. It is essential to seek legal advice immediately. The hearing is an inquiry into the facts as to who the deceased was, and how, when and where he came by his death. The most usual verdicts in a child death due to abuse or neglect are unlawful killing, open verdict, or accident/misadventure. The Coroner will not make any determination of civil (negligence) or criminal liability but an inquest can raise difficult issues for healthcare staff involved in the care of the child as to how the child died.

Part 8 reviews

When a child dies and abuse or neglect are known or suspected, the Area Child Protection Committee will carry out a review to examine whether more could have been done to prevent the tragedy, and how better cooperation between agencies or other measures might prevent a future death. A review will also be considered when a child has sustained life-threatening injury through abuse or neglect, serious sexual abuse or sustained serious impairment of health or development through abuse or neglect. Proposals for review must be discussed with the prosecuting authorities so possible criminal proceedings are not prejudiced. Healthcare professional are under a duty to cooperate with providing information and reports and the advice of the designated professionals should be sought.

Public Inquiries

These may be held, for example, following a series of misdiagnoses of child sex abuse or of widespread institutional abuse. Any health professional who is asked to give evidence should take immediate managerial and legal advice.

Case Scenario

A 2-year-old child presents with bruising to the side of her face which her mother says has been caused by running into a wall while out playing. You suspect that the bruising may be non-accidental. You remember her mother telling you some months earlier that her partner is violent though she denied that he ever touched her daughter. On that previous occasion she forbade you to tell anyone and refused to take your advice to go to social services and/or the police. What do you do?

Clearly it is a matter of clinical judgment as to whether there has been abuse and non-accidental injury may be only one of several possibilities in reaching a diagnosis. To assist you:

- Check the Child Protection Register
- Check the child's medical records to see if there are any previous medical, health visitor or Accident and Emergency reports of similar injuries.

Option 1

You believe that you have clinical grounds for suspecting abuse and are of the opinion that the child is at risk of suffering serious harm but are unsure how to proceed:

- Discuss your concerns with designated senior child protection professional within your health authority. This will be a senior hospital paediatrician and/or a senior nurse with a health visiting qualification (normally based in The Primary Care or National Health Service Trust).
- If clinically indicated and time and circumstances allow, refer the child to a consultant paediatrician.
- Discuss your concerns with the mother and tell her that you intend to inform social services. Tell her that you consider it relevant to share the confidential information which she has given you about her partner's violence towards her with social services, provided it is your opinion that you will not be putting the child at risk of serious harm by doing so. If you think there is a risk, then do not tell the mother what you are going to do.
- Report your concerns verbally to social services and then confirm in writing, making sure to record the name of the social worker.
- Keep copies of the correspondence in the patient's notes.
- Your report should lead to the local authority making S.47 enquiries which should be completed within 7 days of your referral, the purpose of which is to determine whether your patient is in fact a child in need. You will probably be asked to give further information and assistance to the local authority during the course of that investigation. This may lead to:
  - No action except perhaps putting the child on the Child Protection Register, or
  - If necessary, emergency Court proceedings for an Emergency Protection Order/ Exclusion Order/police removal of the child.

If there are long term concerns but social services feel that there is no need for immediate action then it may apply to the Court for:

a S.43 Child Assessment Order

a Care Order

a Supervision Order.

Your input will be vital whichever course of action is taken to attend case conferences, planning meetings in relation to a care order, writing reports and giving evidence in Court if necessary.

Option 2

The mother says she does not know how the bruising occurred and you conclude that it is accidental and the child is not at risk of significant harm. Later it turns out that you were wrong and the child suffers serious injuries as a result of further physical abuse. The consequences may be:

♦ An action by the mother on behalf of the child in negligence in that you failed to meet the standard of care of the ordinary skilled GP by not diagnosing non-accidental bruising or failed to obtain a second opinion from a paediatrician;

♦ a complaint by the mother to the GMC, but this is unlikely to succeed.

References

Bolam v Friern Hospital Management Committee [1957] 1 WLR 582

Bolitho v City and Hackney Health Authority [1997] 4 All ER 771

Gillick v Norfolk Health Authority [1987] 3 All ER 402

In Re C (Adult : Refusal of Treatment) [1994] WLR 290

Re MB (Medical Treatment) [1997] 2FLR 426

Stephens v Avery [1988] 2 All ER 477

Recommended reading

Blumenthal I (1994) *Child Abuse A Handbook for Healthcare Practitioners*. London: Edward Arnold.

British Medical Association (2001) *Consent, rights and choices in health care for children and young people*. London: BMJ BOOKS.

BMA, GMSC, HEA, Brook Advisory Centres, FPA and RCGP (1993) *Confidentiality and People under 16*. London: BMA.

Children Act 1989. London: HMSO.

Department of Health (1999) *Working Together to Safeguard Children*. London: HMSO.

Department of Health (2000) *Framework for the Assessment of Children in Need and their Families*. London: HMSO.

Department of Health: *Good Practice in Consent*, HSC 2001/023. London: HMSO.

Department of Health (2000) *Domestic Violence: A Resource Manual for Health Care Professionals*. London: HMSO.

Department of Health (1996) *The Protection and Use of Patient Information*. London: HMSO.

Department of Health (1992) *Child Protection: Guidance for Senior Nurses, Health Visitors and Midwives*. London: HMSO.

General Medical Council (1999) *Seeking Patients' Consent: The Ethical Considerations*. London: GMC.

General Medical Council (2000) *Confidentiality: Protecting and Providing Information*. London: GMC.

General Medical Council (1997) *A Problem with your Doctor? How the GMC Deals With Complaints*. London: GMC.

General Medical Council (1997) *Facing a Complaint – The GMC's Conduct Procedures*. London: GMC.

Hendrick J (1993) *Child Care for Health Professionals* Abingdon, Oxon OX14 1AA: Radcliffe Medical Press Limited:

Kennedy I and Grubb A (eds) *Medical Law Review.* Oxford: Oxford University Press.

Kennedy I and Grubb A (eds) (1998) *Principles of Medical Law.* Oxford: Oxford University Press.

Marquand P (2000) *Introduction to Medical Law.* Butterworth Heinemann.

Meadow R (ed.) (1997) *ABC of Child Abuse.* London: BMJ Publishing Group.

NHS Executive (1999) *Consent to Treatment – Summary of Legal Rulings,* HSC 1999/03. London: HMSO.

Royal College of Paediatrics and Child Health (1997) *Withholding Or Withdrawing Life-Saving Treatment in Children.* London: RCPCH.

United Kingdom Central Council for Nursing, Midwifery and Health Visiting (1998) *Guidelines for Records and Record Keeping.* London: UKCC.

Chapter 13

Roles and responsibilities

Enid Hendry

Introduction

Working Together to Safeguard Children (Department of Health *et al.* 1999) makes it clear that safeguarding children from harm is everyone's responsibility, and not simply an issue for professionals. This is an important shift in thinking and reflects the view expressed so memorably by Hilary Clinton, that to bring up a child requires a whole village. However, there are specific responsibilities, spelt out in statute and in guidance, that rest with three public sector agencies in particular: the social services, health services and the police. Other statutory and voluntary agencies and professional groups also play important roles in the prevention of abuse and the protection of children, and together form a protective network for the most vulnerable children. When this protective network is functioning effectively it can provide a vital safety net for children, preventing abuse and triggering early responses to concerns.

Individual children need (A) coordinated help from all those who are in contact with them and with their parents and carers, when they are experiencing or are at risk of neglect or abuse.

This requires (B) constructive relationships between different practitioners and a willingness to work with one another. The essential prerequisites for effective partnership working are (C) an appreciation of which groups have a role to play in protecting children and just what are their roles and responsibilities. There is a need to understand what it is reasonable to expect of one another and what is beyond the remit and capacity of different professions and agencies. A is unlikely if B and C are not in place.

This chapter begins by providing an overview of the professional network and the different child protection functions. This is followed by a description of the roles of key professional groups and their main responsibilities in protecting children and preventing their abuse. It concludes by describing the remit of the Area Child Protection Committee, the body charged with ensuring different agencies work together effectively in order to protect children.

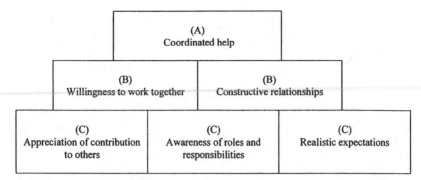

Figure 13.1

Key source documents

Child protection responsibilities are defined in a number of key documents, which are referred to throughout this chapter These are:

- *Working Together to Safeguard Children: A Guide to Inter-agency Working to Safeguard and Promote the Welfare of Children* (Department of Health *et al.* 1999).

- *Framework for the Assessment of Children in Need and their Families* (Department of Health *et al.* 2000).

- *Child Protection – Medical Responsibilities – Guidance to doctors working with Child Protection Agencies: Addendum to Working Together under the Children Act 1989* (Department of Health 1995).

An overview of the professional network

The following diagram, reproduced from *Training Together to Safeguard Children* (NSPCC 2000), represents the groups that together form the inter-agency network. They are grouped as an inner, middle and outer circle, to reflect the extent and frequency of the different professionals' involvement in child protection. This should not be taken to imply that any group gives child protection a low priority or that when they are involved their contribution is of less value than that of others. The boundaries between the circles are permeable and not fixed and will vary at different stages of the child protection process and for different children and families.

> With the exception of the NSPCC, child protection is not the sole purpose of any of the agencies in the network, and numerically, children on the child protection register are a small proportion of the total workload of those agencies. The various agencies have primary commitments which may pull them in very different directions, both in terms of work volume and in terms of values.
>
> Birchall and Hallett (1995 p. 125)

It is important to be mindful of the primary roles of different agencies, when considering their particular child protection responsibilities, as this affects the way these are interpreted and enacted. For instance, a primary concern with crime will mean

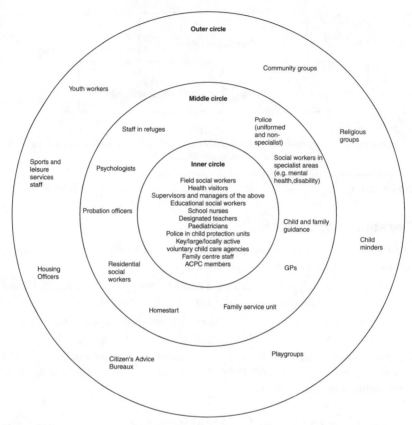

Figure 13.2

police have a particular concern for the preservation of evidence when dealing with suspected child abuse.

Different child protection functions

Within this professional network, groups are likely to be involved in one or more aspect of child protection. Distinct child protection functions can be described as follows:

- The promotion of children's health and welfare and the prevention of abuse
- The identification and reporting of concerns
- The assessment and investigation of concerns about significant harm
- Decision-making and planning
- Taking protective action, including legal action
- Monitoring progress in children and families where there are concerns
- Providing therapeutic and supportive services following the identification of abuse.

The professionals involved in a Section 47 inquiry or in investigative interviews are likely to be different from those involved in the continuing care of abused children. The particular form and nature of the abuse will also affect who is involved, for example:

> The continuing caring network for a teenage victim of a sex ring is likely to need significantly different membership from that needed by a brain damaged baby placed in a permanent substitute family or a neglected toddler of a severely overstressed single parent.
>
> Birchall and Hallett (1995 p. 129)

However, underpinning all of these different roles are some common responsibilities, which cross professional groups. These include:

- Working with parents and children in an open and honest way and wherever possible with their consent and knowledge, except where this would put a child at risk;
- Keeping accurate, signed and dated records of contact with children and families where there are concerns about abuse;
- Sharing information with others in the child protection network when this is necessary to prevent a child suffering significant harm;
- Planning with others how best to intervene in a family;
- Cooperating in the provision of services.

Health professionals

Health professionals play an important part not only with respect to the health of children, but also in relation to their general well being and development.

> Because of the universal nature of health provision, health professionals are often the first to become aware of the needs of children or that some families are experiencing difficulties looking after their children. They should consider what help would benefit those families.
>
> Department of Health (2000, para. 5.21 page 67)

General Practitioners

Their involvement with children and families over long periods of time means that GPs are well placed to recognize when a child is in need of extra help to protect their health and development, or to identify when they are at risk of significant harm. GPs involved in child health surveillance programmes are particularly well situated to identify early indications that a child's development is being adversely affected as a result of the quality of the care they are receiving. The recently introduced *Framework for the Assessment of Children in Need* (Department of Health *et al.* 1999) makes it clear that the GPs role is not simply to refer children to the social services when they suspect actual abuse, but encompasses referring children who are potentially children in need, so that they can be assessed and provided with help in order to prevent future harm. This is entirely consistent with the GPs general duty to maintain the health of their patients, but may not currently be common practice.

In the past GPs may have been worried that a referral to social services for help and support for a family who are experiencing difficulties, might trigger an investigative response involving the police, but little in the way of help. They will have weighed up carefully whether the benefits of making a referral outweigh the potential damage caused. The *Assessment Framework* guidance makes it clear that social services should assess the needs of children and families where it is believed a child is in need, and based on that assessment should ensure the family is provided with services to prevent the child's health and development being impaired. It is only where significant harm is suspected that an investigative response will be triggered.

If GPs have concerns that the problems being experienced by one of their adult patients are placing a child at risk, they have a responsibility to act and to inform social services so that an assessment of the situation can be carried out. This may, for example, be the case where a parent has a mental health problem that is affecting their capacity to respond to a child's essential needs, or where drug or alcohol abuse are seriously impairing the day-to-day functioning of the person concerned. This may present a conflict of interest between the needs of the adult patient and those of the child, but guidance is clear that where there is a risk of significant harm to a child it is their welfare that is the paramount consideration. In many instances it will be appropriate to inform the patient concerned that a referral is being made, however there will be instances where to do so would put a child at increased risk of harm. Situations involving domestic violence can be particularly tricky, as the highest risk of violence to women and children is known to occur when help is sought.

GPs are not usually directly involved in the investigation of abuse, but they may have a significant contribution to make in relation to initial and core assessments of children who are thought to be in need of protection. They are likely to be consulted by social services staff when referrals are received which involve concerns about a child's welfare or safety. The medical history of a child who is thought to be suffering as a result of neglect can form a crucial part of an assessment. When a non-accidental injury is suspected, information on whether a child has been brought for treatment, if so, what explanation was given, what was the demeanour of the parent and child and what was the GPs view of the injury, will all form an important contribution to an assessment of what happened.

GPs can also contribute to making decisions on whether a child is at continuing risk of abuse and should consequently have their name placed on the child protection register. To do so it is important to participate in the initial child protection conference. Ideally GPs should attend the conference, but where this is not possible there are other ways of contributing, through, for example, written reports or prior discussion with the conference Chair. This will always be a second best, as it is only by being present that other perspectives and information can build up a picture which allows the most appropriate decisions to be made.

Although the numbers of abused children seen by a GP may be relatively small, GPs are likely to be involved in the ongoing medical treatment of some children who have been abused. For example, a child who has been sexually abused may become anorexic or may experience post-traumatic stress disorder and related problems. While a doctor's primary focus may not be the abuse per se, there is obviously a need to understand the impact of abuse in planning treatment and to consider what is currently happening to the person concerned. Is there a reoccurrence of the abuse? Is there a court case in connection with the abuse that is causing stress and anxiety?

Ongoing monitoring of children who have been identified as at risk of abuse is another area of responsibility. GPs need to ensure that patient records are marked in such a way that they can be alerted to children whose names are on the child protection register, and any cause for renewed concern must be reported promptly so that if necessary it can be looked into by the key worker for the child.

It is clear then that GPs have a role and contribution to make to many aspects and stages of the child protection process. They can only play this role if they remain alert to the possibility of abuse and ready to act where necessary in children's best interests.

Paediatricians

While abused children form a small proportion of the patients seen by community and hospital-based paediatricians, child abuse has become a very significant part of their workload. They should be alert to the possibility of abuse in relation to all the children with whom they are involved and know how to act on any concerns. However, they are most likely to be involved in child protection work when concerns about a child's health and development or abuse are referred to them for a medical assessment. The assessment of even relatively minor injuries in children is important, as there may be evidence of other previously undisclosed injuries, such as broken bones. Differential diagnoses may be required in relation to physical injuries, sexual abuse, neglect or emotional abuse.

Paediatricians may be asked to contribute to an assessment of a child, both in cases where they are already involved with a child or in cases where expert opinion is needed on some aspect of the child's health or development or on injuries they have sustained. This may be, for example, where a child is failing to thrive and the cause is uncertain. It may be in relation to a disabled child where there is concern that delayed development or behavioural problems are not attributable to the child's impairment but rather to parental care or the lack of it. The paediatrician's view on the causes of developmental delay may be critical to the outcome of an assessment and to the decision of the child protection conference.

They may also be asked to advise in cases of suspected sexual abuse, for instance, where there are physical signs that could have different explanations or causes. Cases such as these were notoriously the source of much difficulty and disagreement in Cleveland in the 1980s. Since then it has been made clear that it is usually unsafe to rely solely on medical diagnosis to determine whether a child has been abused and that a comprehensive assessment, of which the medical assessment is one aspect, is what is needed.

In addition to contributing to assessments and investigations paediatricians may also be required to give a medical opinion in civil and criminal court.

A doctor is able to present the factual and clinical findings and, if able to justify a claim to be an expert witness, he may also present medical opinion as evidence. The extent of his clinical expertise will obviously affect the weight which is given to any expert evidence. This emphasizes the value of making the initial referral to a consultant paediatrician or other doctor with specialist expertise an experience.

Jones et al. (1987 p. 128.)

Paediatricians also have a part to play in the ongoing management, monitoring and treatment of children who have been abused and neglected.

Each Health Authority will identify a senior paediatrician to take the professional lead on child protection and to act as a source of advice and training on child protection matters, not just within the health service but also for the wider local network. This person is usually a member of the Area Child Protection Committee.

Health visitors, midwives and school nurses

'Nurses work in a variety of settings where they are likely to meet vulnerable children and their families' (Department of Health *et al.* 1999). This means they are well placed to identify and report concerns both about a child's health and welfare and about actual abuse. Whatever their work context, they should have the skills and confidence to act promptly on concerns, to share information appropriately and to contribute to assessments. School nurses monitor children's health and development routinely, and are well placed to identify and discuss concerns with young people and if necessary to refer to others.

The *Framework for the Assessment of Children in Need* (Department of Health 2000) describes the midwife and health visitor as

> Uniquely well placed to identify risk factors to a child during pregnancy, birth, and the child's early care. Health visitors and school nurses monitor child health, growth and physical, emotional and social development. In addition, health visitors are aware of the health of the parents and may identify particular difficulties, for example post-natal depression in mothers.

Their role is therefore concerned with:

- The promotion of children's health and welfare;
- The prevention of abuse, through providing advice and support to parents and through early identification of difficulties;
- Recognition and reporting of concerns, wherever possible with the consent of the parent concerned, unless this would put the child at greater risk;
- Contributing to initial and core assessments;
- Contributing to the analysis of information, for example at child protection conferences, and helping to make professional judgements, decisions and plans, possibly as a member of a core group;
- Monitoring progress in families where there are concerns or where a child's name has been placed on the register;
- Providing advice and support to parents who have neglected or abused their children.

It will be apparent from the above list that their role is both broad and challenging, and balances preventive and remedial functions. Given the size of their caseloads it is important to be realistic about what they can and cannot be expected to do with families, and to clarify the boundaries between their roles and that of the social worker. It may be tempting to rely heavily on the health visitor where they are the only professional who has access to a family, but this may place an unfair burden on the health visitor.

Health visitors have a key role to play in relation to child neglect, and in recognizing when it has become so serious that it is significantly impairing a child's development. They need to be able to present their assessment and professional opinion to colleagues in the professional network in a way that ensures they are listened to and that timely action is taken. This means being assertive, persistent and evidence based. All too often children have been left for too long in situations of appalling neglect because the concerns of health visitors have not been taken seriously or given due weight.

Social workers

Social workers in the local authority and the NSPCC have statutory responsibilities for child protection. Social services departments have a duty to safeguard and promote the welfare of children in their area who are in need, to promote the upbringing of such children by their parents, provided that is consistent with their welfare, and to provide services to support families. They are expected to fulfil these responsibilities by work in partnership with parents and with other agencies. They also have a duty to 'make enquiries,' under Section 47 of the Children Act 1989, if they believe a child in their area is suffering or is likely to suffer significant harm. This will usually be done with the police. On the basis of these inquiries they are expected to take whatever action is needed, in partnership with others, to safeguard the child from harm.

Where a child is considered by a child protection conference to be at continuing risk of significant harm the social services department is responsible for coordinating an inter-agency plan, based on an assessment of need, and for its implementation and periodic review. They may find it necessary to apply to the court for an Emergency Protection Order, which will place a child under their protection for a maximum of eight days. In more persistent or serious cases, they may apply to court for a Care Order, and if successful may place the child with foster carers or in residential care.

In most situations of child abuse this does not prove to be necessary, as most abused children remain with one or both parent. It is no longer possible for social workers to remove a child from his or her parents without the approval of a court.

It will be apparent that social services departments carry both caring/supportive roles and controlling/authority roles in relation to parents and their children. These functions are exercised on their behalf by social workers, who have to be able to contain the inherent tensions and dilemmas this creates in their day to day work with families.

Social workers work in a variety of settings, which determine what is their particular role and contribution to the protection of children. For example, social workers working in residential settings will be primarily concerned with the care of children and young people and with their health and welfare. A significant proportion of young people in residential care have experienced abuse and therefore the social workers have a role in providing advice, support and counselling. Regrettably, while some of the most needy young people are placed in residential care, the staff working with them tend to be the least well qualified and trained group of social workers. Residential social workers also need to remain alert to the possibility of abuse occurring within the home, as abuse has become a widely recognized feature of residential care. Abuse may be by peers or by members of staff. It may be current or historical. Blowing the whistle on colleagues or making a judgement that sexual activity between peers is not consensual and may constitute abuse both require considerable confidence and courage from residential workers.

Field social workers in duty or intake teams will be responsible for receiving and responding to referrals or requests for help from families themselves and from professionals. They have to decide on the basis of the information received, whether it appears that a child is in need or at risk of significant harm. To ascertain this they will usually need to gather and analyse information from a range of sources, including the child or young person and other family members, as well as from the professional network. A decision on a course of action has to be made within 24 hours of a referral. This will usually follow discussion with other members of the professional network.

If it is thought that a child may be at risk of significant harm or be a child in need the social worker's role is to ensure an initial assessment is carried out, covering the areas identified in the *Framework for the Assessment of Children in Need* (Department of Health *et al.* 2000). They have to gather and evaluate information on each child's developmental needs, the parents' capacity to respond to those needs and the family history and key environmental factors. If abuse is suspected they must also carry out a section 47 inquiry with the police and medical experts, as necessary, to find out what has happened and what action is needed to safeguard any child at risk of significant harm. In practical terms this may mean making contact with and gaining the cooperation of parents and children, as well as speaking to any number of professionals who also know the family. It will involve weighing and evaluating complex and often incomplete information, often in the face of considerable pressure and anxiety from other professionals and from parents, sometimes in the face of violence directed at the worker. Social workers will usually form their assessment in consultation with a more senior member of staff. If it appears that a criminal prosecution may be required, then the social worker will carry out a video recorded investigative interview of the child witness with the police.

The social worker's continuing responsibilities include:

♦ convening an initial child protection conference

♦ preparing the young person and family members for the child protection conference

♦ preparing and presenting a report to the conference

♦ being a member of the core group, responsible for developing the action plan following the conference

♦ carrying out a core assessment, with contributions from others

- working with the young person and with family members to reduce the risk of continuing significant harm
- helping the young person recover from the effects of abuse
- monitoring progress
- preparing and presenting evidence in court where problems prove intractable.

These different roles may be carried out by different social workers, as it is not unusual for social services departments to transfer cases needing longer term involvement after an initial assessment.

Police

The police have dual responsibilities for protecting life and for preventing crime. Child abuse straddles their role to detect and control crime and their civil responsibilities for crime prevention and public protection. Their role in terms of contributing to the overall well-being of children is recognized in the *Assessment Framework* (p. 77), which encourages them to make information available to social services that could help in a 'child in need' assessment, based on their knowledge of local communities and families. This may be particularly relevant, for example, when called out to incidents of domestic violence where a child is a member of the household. There is a strong interrelationship between domestic violence and the abuse of children, and the police may be the only agency to be aware of a level of violence which is escalating or threatening a child.

While this contribution to safeguarding children is important, the primary child protection role and responsibility of the police is to investigate suspected criminal offences committed against children. The nature of child abuse means that in some, but not all, cases this leads to the apprehension and charging of the offender. All police forces now have specialist child protection units, which investigate all aspects of child abuse in families and institutions. This has enabled the police to select staff who are suited to this sensitive area of work and to provide them with specialist training. These officers work closely with social workers to ascertain what has happened, to gather information to assess how to best to intervene and, where appropriate, to gather evidence which may be used in a criminal prosecution. Where it is necessary to gather evidence for a criminal prosecution, the police and social worker may carry out an investigative interview with a child which they video record, for future use in court. Only specially trained staff can carry out these video recorded interviews.

While social workers and police in most parts of the country have developed excellent working relationships to protect children, there are tensions between their roles and primary focus that have to be managed and negotiated. The police role is primarily one of law enforcement, while the social work focus is child welfare. The two can pull in opposite directions at times, causing strains in relationships and disagreements about how to intervene. For example, early morning raids on family homes where sexual abuse is suspected, have been carried out in order to maximize the chances of preserving evidence. This may be seriously detrimental to future working relationships with non-abusing family members and also extremely distressing to the children concerned.

Social workers have to continue working in partnership with parents in the interests of children, while this is not necessary for the police.

The police should be informed as soon as there is reason to believe a crime may have been committed against a child, and a strategy discussion will allow the necessary planning of how to proceed to take place. While their involvement in cases of physical abuse and sexual abuse is relatively clear cut, it may be less clear whether and if so how they should be involved in cases of neglect and emotional abuse. This will depend in part on the nature and severity of the case.

The police are uniquely empowered to enter premises in an emergency, and to ensure the immediate protection of children believed to be suffering significant harm through the use of police protection powers. These will only be used where it is not possible to seek an Emergency Protection Order. They have also been given the responsibility for coordinating and leading the risk assessment and management process for the exchange of information about people who have been convicted of a sexual offence and who are believed to pose a risk to children.

The police are also responsible for initiating, but not for conducting, criminal proceedings. They are required to consider whether there is sufficient evidence to prosecute, whether it is in the public interest and whether it is in the best interest of the child. This latter consideration should be based on consultation with partner agencies and with the child themselves, if they are of an age and ability to influence the decision.

Area Child Protection Committees (ACPC)

Originally known as Area Review Committees, the ACPC role and remit is set out in *Working Together to Safeguard Children* (Department of Health *et al.* 1999). It is an inter-agency forum for agreeing how the different services and professional groups should cooperate to safeguard children in each Local Authority area. The ACPC is charged with making sure arrangements work effectively in the interests of children. They do this by:

- Publishing policies and procedures for inter-agency child protection work. All professionals should ensure they have access to and comply with these inter-agency procedures.

- Ensuring that there are local opportunities for training on child protection, including training on inter-agency working. They usually have a Training Sub Committee, which organizes a comprehensive programme of inter-agency training open to member agencies.

- Undertaking case reviews, known as Part 8 reviews, when a child dies or in the event of serious cases of abuse. This includes making sure the findings from such reviews are understood, communicated and acted upon.

- Quality assuring and auditing child protection practice, for example through case audits.

- Ensuring agreements and understanding across agencies of what is meant by abuse and when a child crosses the 'significant harm' threshold.

- Raising awareness within the wider community of the need to safeguard children.
- Publishing an annual business plan.

ACPCs should have members from each of the main agencies responsible for protecting children, and they should be sufficiently senior to be able to take decisions. Health Services are usually represented by a designated doctor and designated nurse and by a Health Authority representative. Identifying someone who can represent GPs in a meaningful way often proves a challenge for ACPCs. Many ACPCs publish newsletters to keep professionals informed about their activities. Details about who chairs and who sits on your local ACPC can be obtained from your local Social Services Department.

Conclusions

There are many other professional groups who can play a role in protecting children – in education, in youth work, in housing and leisure services, and in day care. Children's lives bring them into contact with many individuals and agencies, all of whom can contribute to their safety and well-being. They have a right to expect of us that we talk to one another, understand each other's roles and work together in a cooperative endeavour to keep them safe.

References

Birchall E and Hallett C (1995) *Working Together in Child Protection*. London: HMSO.

Department of Health (1995) *Child Protection – Medical Responsibilities*. London: The Stationery Office.

Department of Health, Department for Education and Employment, Home Office and the National Assembly for Wales (1999) *Working Together to Safeguard Children*. London: The Stationery Office.

Department of Health, Department for Education and Employment, Home Office (2000) *Framework for the Assessment of Children in Need and their Families*. London: The Stationery Office.

Jones D, Pickett J, Oates M and Barbor P (1987) *Understanding Child Abuse*, 2nd edn. London: Macmillan Education.

Chapter 14

Ethics and the child protection process

Anne-Marie Slowther

Introduction

The area of child protection is challenging, and at times disturbing, for the general practitioner. The evidence on which to base a diagnosis, or suspicion of child abuse is often not as clear-cut as that involved in physical or even psychological disorders. The doctor's core relationship with her individual patient may be in conflict with her role as a member of a multi-agency team in which she is not the principal decision-maker. Her role as a family doctor means that she may have conflicting responsibilities to different members of the same family, all of whom are her patients. In addition, her duties to the wider public, and her legal duties, may be in conflict with what her individual patients' want, and indeed with what she feels would be in their best interests. Although these issues occur in many aspects of a GP's work, they are thrown into sharp relief in all stages of the child protection process: prevention, diagnosis, reporting and management. How can a GP resolve these conflicting moral values?

The legal framework

Unlike many areas of health care, child protection does have a statutory legal framework (The Children Act 1989) within which health care practitioners must operate. There are also guidelines produced by Area Child Protection Committees for use by local practitioners. The legal aspects of child protection are discussed in detail elsewhere in this book so I shall not discuss this further, except to highlight two consequences of the presence of legislation in this area. First, in considering the ethical issues surrounding a possible case of child abuse, a GP must be aware of her legal obligations; and second, the ethical principles underlying the law provide us with some idea of the weight society gives to the conflicting moral values inherent in this area. The underlying moral value in the Children Act is that the interests of the child, and of children in general, are paramount. However, the existence of legislation in this area does not mean that the ethical dilemmas have been removed. The law needs to be interpreted in the context of an individual case, and many cases are not clear-cut.

The guidance for doctors working with child protection agencies (Department of Health 1995) talks about a 'critical threshold of professional concern' needing to be reached before referral to the statutory agencies for child protection. It states that the critical threshold of professional concern is 'a matter of individual professional judgement made by someone with experience in child protection matters and will invariably vary between professionals and between situations'.

Even when there is no doubt that a referral is required, there are still ethical considerations around how the referral and subsequent management of the case are handled to ensure that the interests of the child are best served while taking into account the interests of other parties in the case.

The moral framework

Several different moral values or principles need to be considered in the child protection process. How much weight is given to each of these, and how they interact with each other, will depend on the facts of a particular case. No one moral principle will provide an answer in every case. However, an awareness of the values involved will facilitate the process of decision-making in such ethically sensitive cases.

Some moral principles

The duty of a doctor to act in her patient's best interests

This duty is traditionally the cornerstone of the doctor-patient relationship. I should not act in a way that will bring harm to my patient, and I should act to bring benefit to my patient. It encapsulates two of the four principles of biomedical ethics expounded by Beauchamp and Childress (1994). In the case of a child whom the GP knows, or strongly suspects, to have been severely physically, emotionally or sexually abused, the duty to act in her patient's best interests will dictate that she refers the child to social services in order to prevent further harm. However, if there is concern that a child may be at risk, but no strong evidence to support this, it will not be clear that referring the child to social services is in his or her best interests. Further consideration of the consequences of the various options will be necessary.

What if the patient sitting in front of the GP in surgery is not the 'at risk' child, but the mother? She expresses concern that her partner is occasionally physically abusing her child but begs the GP not to say anything because if her partner finds out she has spoken to someone, he will become even more violent towards her. The duty to act in her patient's best interests would suggest that the GP should respect the mother's request for confidentiality. The child may not be a patient of the GP and if so, there would be no duty of care in the context of a doctor-patient relationship between the GP and the child.

Maximizing the good

The concept of maximizing the good comes from John Stuart Mill's theory of utilitarianism (1962 [1863]). This is a form of consequentialism where the moral worth of an action is judged by the consequences of that action. In utilitarianism, the morally correct action is the one that produces the most 'utility' or 'good' as its consequence. This moral principle has several implications for decision-making in the context of child protection.

1 When considering what course of action would be in the child's best interests, it is usually necessary to evaluate as far as possible the consequences to that child of the various options. This will include the consequences of initiating a full investigation of a family when there is a suspicion of child abuse, which is ultimately found to be incorrect, as well as the consequences of failing to refer in a case and thus allowing the abuse to continue.

2 The implications of a GP's action for the rest of the family, who may also be the GP's patients, are also worthy of consideration. If the family falls apart under the scrutiny of an investigation this may affect the health and well-being of the child at risk, and so not be in his or her best interests. It could also affect the health and well-being of other members of the family resulting in a 'less good' situation for the whole family. However, the consequences of failing to recognize and report abuse may mean that the continuing abuse itself destroys the family, or that other children in the family also become victims. Which action will produce maximum benefit for the whole family?

3 The consequence of the action on society is also a consideration in child protection. Not reporting suspected abuse could mean that an abuser would be able to abuse many children, not just those in a single family. The concept of the public interest, which may override an individual's interests, suggests that the consequences of a doctor's actions on the wider community are an important moral consideration. I have already suggested that the law on this issue reflects society's belief that in this area the best interests of the child are paramount. Therefore, if it became clear that doctors were not disclosing information about suspected abuse because of concerns about, for example, breaching confidentiality, the loss of faith in the medical profession by the public in this area could lead to a wider distrust of doctors with detrimental effects on health care.

Respect for autonomy

Respect for autonomy has become a powerful moral principle in western medicine over recent years. Many people would now consider it the most important moral principle governing the doctor–patient relationship. It is another of the four principles of biomedical ethics listed by Beauchamp and Childress (1994). An autonomous person should be able to make choices, free from coercion, that are consistent with how she wishes to live her life. The principle of respect for patients' autonomy has several implications for health care. Perhaps the most obvious is that patients should be provided with information and explanation to allow them to make a choice about their treatment. This is the basis of informed consent. Another area where the principle of respect for autonomy impacts on health care is confidentiality. It is generally accepted in our society that doctors have a duty to protect patient confidentiality, and it has been recognized by the courts that it is in the public interest that this should be so. If a patient gives a doctor information during a consultation, expecting that the information will be treated confidentially, and the doctor then passes that information to a third party, the patient's choice to keep the information confidential has been overridden. His or her autonomy has been compromised. To justify overriding a patient's autonomy in this way, a doctor would need a strong moral, or legal, justification. An example would be the prevention of harm to another person, or detrimental consequences for society.

The autonomy of children should also be respected. If a child can understand and evaluate the choices involved in a particular course of treatment then their autonomous consent to, or request for, treatment should be respected. This principle was upheld in English law in the case of provision of contraception to girls younger than sixteen (Gillick 1995). Similarly, if a child fully understands the implications of confidentiality in a particular situation, and states that they wish information to remain confidential, their autonomy should be respected and confidentiality maintained. Breach of confidentiality could be justified as in the case of an adult, by the need to protect others. However, with an adult we would not override a person's autonomy to protect them, rather than others, from harm, for example if an adult refused beneficial treatment we would respect their decision. In the case of a child, we do sometimes override their autonomous decision in order to protect them from harm or to act in their best interests. This view is supported by the English courts (Re: W 1992).

Virtue ethics

Virtue ethics is a moral theory that does not rely on principles or rules, but considers moral behaviour in terms of the virtues exhibited by the moral agent (that is the person making the moral decision). It has its origins in the writings of Aristotle, but has been elaborated on by more recent philosophers. It does not lend itself so easily to directing how a person should behave in a particular situation, but it emphasizes the need to develop characteristics that enable a person to make the morally right decision. In the context of child abuse, doctors will need to cultivate virtues such as courage and wisdom in order to steer a path through an area fraught with difficulty and with no easy answers.

Moral decision-making

A knowledge of the different moral values and principles that underlie the child protection process does not, in itself, provide an answer to the question of what a GP should do in a particular situation. It is necessary to consider the weight of each value in the particular situation, given the facts of the individual case. In many cases, the facts will be so clear that there is no doubt about what is the morally correct course of action, and this is likely to be reinforced by a legal duty. If there is a definite allegation, or unequivocal signs of abuse, then protecting the child from harm is of paramount importance. However, in grey areas where there is suspicion only, it may be necessary to consider the ethical implications of the situation more carefully. How can a GP use her knowledge of the relevant moral principles, and of the facts of the case, to come to an appropriate decision?

We do not make decisions in a moral vacuum. An individual GP will bring to any decision her own moral values and an awareness of the moral position of the profession on this issue. There may be professional guidelines on specific issues, such as the General Medical Council's guidelines on confidentiality (GMC 2000). Legislation may dictate what must be done or provide guidance on balancing the conflicting values in a particular situation. Discussion with colleagues, if necessary using anonymised information, can sometimes help to clarify arguments.

A useful framework to consider the ethical issues in clinical decision-making has been developed by Schneider and Snell (2000). This approach, which has the acronym CARE, identifies four key areas to consider in approaching an ethical issue.

1 The Core moral values of the decision-maker.

2 The previous Actions of the decision-maker in similar situations.

3 The Reasoned opinions of others about similar situations.

4 The actions or Experiences of others when faced with similar situations.

These can be used in the context of a GP considering the ethical issues in a case of suspected abuse. How the GP has behaved previously in similar circumstances, and how they feel about their previous actions, will influence the decision. The reasoned opinions of others would include professional and legal guidelines. The previous experience of others may include published cases, or previous cases in the practice.

Theory into practice

Ethical considerations in diagnosis and reporting of alleged or suspected abuse

Hypothetical case scenario A

The mother of a thirteen-year-old girl attends her GP's surgery with symptoms of anxiety and depression. She has been a frequent attender at the surgery over several years with psychological problems, but has recently remarried and has been much happier and more settled since then. During the consultation, she says that her daughter has told her that her stepfather has, on two or three occasions when the mother was not in the house, attempted to kiss her and touch her breasts. Confronted by the mother, the stepfather has admitted his behaviour but said that he is ashamed of what he has done and that it won't happen again. The mother is afraid that if social services become involved she will not be able to cope with the resulting stress and will become severely depressed again. The following day the girl, an articulate and self-confident child, attends the surgery with her mother and states that she does not want the authorities to be told because they might break up the family. She is still fond of her stepfather and realizes that he is a stabilizing and positive influence on her mother. In general, the family has been much happier since he became a part of it. The girl has two younger sisters.

Hypothetical case scenario B

A thirty-year-old woman attends surgery with a black eye and bruising on her arms. In response to questioning by the GP, she admits that her husband has hit her, and that this has happened before. She says that her husband has a fiery temper, especially when he has been drinking. The GP recalls seeing the woman's five-year-old son in the surgery two or three times in the past couple of months. He has been investigated for a urinary tract infection after wetting his bed on a few occasions, and two consultations have been for minor injuries said to have been sustained in the school playground. For these latter consultations, he was brought to the surgery by his father, the woman's husband. The GP asks the mother if there is any possibility that her husband is hitting his son as well as her. She flatly denies this, and also denies that her son has ever seen her being hit. She insists that she does not want details of her marital abuse to be divulged to anyone else.

These two case scenarios illustrate some of the ethical issues that can arise in the child protection process.

1   The best interests of the child are of prime importance, but it may not be clear whether their best interests will be served by reporting the alleged or suspected abuse.

2   There will be consequences either way for other family members. In scenario A, reporting the abuse may disrupt the family, precipitate a depressive illness in the mother and result in her being unable to care for her children. If the abuse is not reported, the stepfather may resume his behaviour with the girl or one of her siblings. In scenario B, if suspected abuse is reported, the woman could suffer further beatings when her husband found out that she had told her GP about his behaviour.

3   In scenario A, there may be consequences for the wider public if the abuse is not reported. The man may have a job that involves supervision of young girls.

4   In scenario B, reporting suspected abuse would mean overriding the mother's autonomy and breaking confidentiality. There would need to be a strong moral justification for this. In scenario A, the girl's autonomy would be compromised by disclosure. The consequence in both cases is likely to be a loss of trust in the GP at the very time when the GP's support of the family could be crucial.

There are no easy answers, but if a GP facing similar situations is able to identify the ethical issues and make a considered judgement, in the light of professional and legal guidelines, she should be able to feel confident that her decision can be morally justified. This does not guarantee that it will be the correct decision in retrospect, but that is a problem that GPs face in many aspects of their clinical decision-making. Unfortunately we do not always get it right.

References

Beauchamp TL and Childress JF (1994) *Principles of Biomedical Ethics.* New York: Oxford University Press.

Children Act (1989) London: HMSO.

Department of Health, British Medical Association, Conference of Royal Medical Colleges (1995) *Child Protection: Medical Responsibilities.*

Gillick *v* West Norfolk & Wisbech AHA [1986] AC 112. [1985] 3 WLR 830.

GMC (2000) *Confidentiality: Protecting and Providing Information.* London: General Medical Council.

Mill JS (1962) Utilitarianism [1863] in M Warnock (ed.) *Utilitarianism: John Stuart Mill.* London: Harper Collins.

Re W (A minor) (Medical treatment: Court's jurisdiction) Fam 64; [1992] 3WLR 758.

Schneider GW and Snell L (2000) C.A.R.E.: an approach for teaching ethics in medicine. *Social Science and Medicine* 51: 1563–7.

Chapter 15

The child protection case conference

Wendy Thorn and Michael J. Bannon

Child protection case conference: purpose

Communication and coordination are fundamental to the entire child protection process. Repeated public inquiries into high profile cases of severe child maltreatment have emphasized the need for effective flows of information between agencies and individual professionals regarding the welfare of individual children (Butler-Sloss 1988; Blom-Cooper 1987). In the UK, the main forum for communication and intervention with respect to the protection of children from abuse is the *Child Protection Case Conference* (CPCC). This represents a multidisciplinary meeting attended by members of a child's family and involved professionals from a number of agencies. The meeting is chaired by a senior professional (usually from Social Services). The chair should have no direct contact with the family and should also be independent of operational or management responsibility of the professional most involved in the case.

The key functions of the CPCC may be summarized as follows:

1   To enable the sharing of information regarding a child's health, development and safety;

2   To determine if a child is at risk of significant harm;

3   To agree upon a plan of action, if appropriate, in order to safeguard a child's welfare.

A decade ago, Gibbons estimated that 40,000 child protection case conferences were convened in England per annum (Gibbons *et al.* 1995).

The CPCC process

Preparation

As shown in Figure 15.1, the CPCC represents a pivotal event in the overall child protection process. As agreement of crucial decisions regarding children's welfare is part of this process, it follows that adequate preparation is undertaken by professionals

160,000 referrals to child protection agencies

⇓

120,000 investigations

⇓

40,000 child protection case conferences

⇓

24,500 additions to child protection registers

Figure 15.1 CPCCs in England, 1992.

prior to the conference itself. The Children Act (1989) defines clearly the purpose and function of the CPCC. Section 47 of the Act places a clear duty upon both professionals and agencies to positively assist Social Services with their enquiries where 'there is reasonable cause to suspect that a child is suffering, or is likely to suffer, significant harm'. The conference should be held within 15 working days of the initial strategy meeting. This usually allows time for some degree of risk assessment to be undertaken. It should also be noted that this 15-day limit is a performance indicator that is actively monitored by the Social Services Inspectorate. The following preparation is undertaken:

1 The family are involved at the earliest possible stage. Social Services discuss with the family who will attend, the purpose of the conference and advice regarding legal issues and advocacy.

2 If appropriate, dependent upon the child's age and level of understanding, s/he will be offered the opportunity to attend and to bring a friend or advocate.

3 It is also the responsibility of Social Services to provide a written report which summarises the information that has been gathered as a result of the initial family assessment and section 47 enquires (if possible). The report is detailed and provides a factual account leading to the present investigation. It takes into account:

   ◆ previous significant events or concerns in the case of the family

   ◆ information on the child's health and development

   ◆ professional opinion on the ability of parents and carers to meet the needs of the child

   ◆ views of parents and child (if appropriate)

   ◆ overall analysis, dependent upon the above, of the child's overall current safety and possible future risk.

Reporting of concerns

⇓

Initial investigation

⇓

Strategy meeting

⇓

Convene case conference

⇓

Risk assessment	Engagement of family	Involvement of professionals	Collation of information

⇓

Child Protection Case Conference (within 15 days of strategic meeting)

⇓

If registered

⇓

Definition of child protection plan	Identification of core group	Appointment of key worker

⇓

Review conferences

⇓

Deregister

Figure 15.2 The Child Protection Case Conference.

All CPCC participants are provided with a copy of this report prior to the meeting.

4 During the conference, attending professionals will be asked to provide details of their particular involvement with the child and family. They are actively encouraged to prepare beforehand a written summary that may be made available at the meeting.

5 Careful consideration is given to the number and type of professional who will be invited to attend. The list will obviously vary with each case but might include:

  ◆ Social Services
  ◆ Foster carers

- Professionals involved with the child:
  GP, Health Visitor, School Nurse, Paediatrician, Teacher
- Professionals involved with the family:
  GP, probation services, adult mental health services
- Police
- Local authority legal advisor

The conference process and protocol

1 The conference chair usually begins by introducing all attendees. The purpose of the conference (as well as possible outcomes) are clearly stated.

2 Time is allowed for the reading of any additional information made available for the conference.

3 Each professional is asked to give his or her contribution in terms of fact and opinion.

4 Similarly, the family and child (if appropriate) will also be asked to contribute.

5 At the end of this process, a decision must be made around whether or not the child is considered to be at continuing risk of significant harm. Every Area Child Protection Committee has written criteria to assist professionals as to whether the criteria for registration have been met. In general, however, the test for registration should be that:

- A child has suffered abuse or neglect; and/or
- is likely to be the subject of further maltreatment in the future.

6 If the answer is yes to either or both of the above, then it is usual for the child's name to be placed on the local child protection register under one of the following categories: *physical, emotional, sexual abuse* or *neglect*. Once a child is registered the following actions are undertaken:

- A *child protection plan* is defined; this identifies the changes needed in order to safeguard the child's welfare and outlines a contingency plan in the event of subsequent adverse developments
- A *key worker* is appointed to the case who has overall responsibility for ensuring that the child protection plan is implemented
- A *core group* of professionals and family members is established who will develop and put into practice the child protection plan.

7 In some instances, while there may be concerns regarding a child's welfare, a decision may be taken not to register and other arrangements will be undertaken.

Post conference events

1 It is agreed good practice that a *core assessment* is undertaken within 42 working days of registration. This assessment includes a description of the child's needs as well as the perceived caring abilities of parents or carers. On occasion, additional

specialist opinion may be commissioned from other agencies such as, for example, child and adolescent mental health professionals, in order to facilitate this process.

2   A written agreement should be produced for parents that outlines the reasons for registration and the purpose and process of the protection plan.

3   The child protection plan is likely to outline a number of practical interventions designed to promote child welfare and positive parenting with agreed timescales. These might include therapy for a child who has been the victim of abuse or counselling for the perpetrator.

4   Child protection review conferences will be held following initial registration (usually within three months) and at intervals for as long as the child's name remains on the register. The format is similar in principle to the initial child protection case conference, but the number of professionals who attend is less and the focus is directed towards continued assessment of risk as well as that of rehabilitation.

5   Removal of a child's name from the register (deregistration) takes place if the child is no longer considered to be at risk or has moved to another authority area. Deregistration also occurs when a child reaches the age of 18 years.

Child protection case conferences and the GP

GPs have much to contribute to the decision making process at conferences in terms of sharing of useful information and assessment of risk:

1   As a result of their participation in child health surveillance programmes, GPs have access to unique knowledge of individual children in terms of their development, physical health and emotional well-being.

2   As GPs provide continuing care for entire families and communities, they can provide a boarder picture of families with respect to their ability to provide care for children; this is of particular relevance when chronic physical ill-health, mental illness, domestic violence and/or alcohol/substance abuse on the part of carers may adversely affect a child's development.

3   They will often have knowledge of local services and avenues of support for dysfunctional families and carers.

4   GPs are well placed to actively participate in the child protection plan by offering support to both children and their carers.

5   It follows that by participating in the sharing of information and concerns, the GP's knowledge of the child and his family will also be enhanced.

Regular statistics are maintained by local Area Child Protection Committees regarding the number of conferences convened, their timing with respect to the initial investigation and attendance by various professional groups. Birchall and Hallett (1995) confirmed that conferences were:

◆ convened after 14 days of the initial investigation

◆ usually held in Social Services premises

- large with more than half of conferences having ten or more attendees
- poorly attended by GPs.

The low attendance rate by GPs at CPCCs has been the subject of concern by Social Services Departments for some years. Simpson et al in 1994 documented GP input to 190 conferences as follows:

No input from GP: 72%
GP sent report only: 18%
GP attended: 9%
GP attended and provided report: 1%

A more recent survey in Nottinghamshire found that GPs attend between 7–14% of conferences (Polnay 2000). It is recognized that GPs undertake an important role in the holistic care of children and their families and are well placed to act as influential advocates on their behalf. Non-attendance and, worse still, lack of provision of reports to conferences has created tension between social workers and GPs. In recognition of the importance of the potential contribution that might be made by GPs at CPCCs, numerous researchers have sought to seek the underlying causes for their poor showing at conferences in the hope that possible solutions might be found.

Early studies were focused upon practical factors that might impair GP attendance (Boyter *et al.* 1983; Lea-Cox and Hall 1991; Bisset and Hunter 1992; Birchall and Hallett 1995). These included:

- Alleged poor timing of conferences which conflicted with booked surgery times;
- Inconvenient location, often on Social Services premises with poor provision for parking;
- Inadequate notice which prevented GPs from making alternative arrangements for booked surgeries;
- Lack of funding for locum cover.

Authors of these studies suggested that attendance by GPs would improve if practical solutions to these barriers were found.

Some researchers have challenged the perception that practical difficulties (timing, venue etc.) alone were responsible for the poor attendance rate by GPs. Hallett in 1995 confirmed low attendance rates by GPs and studied the notice given for conferences as well as their venue. She found that few conferences were convened in less than two weeks from the initial investigation, the implication being that at least ten days notice would be given to attendees.

Bannon *et al.* (1997) convened five focus groups among primary health care teams in the West Midlands in 1995 to determine their views regarding their input into the child protection process. The groups consisted of mainly primary health care team staff but on occasion, social workers as well. Divergent views regarding case conferences were evident with respect to perceptions held by GPs and social workers.

In general GPs were reluctant to attend conferences on the basis that they had little to contribute and that attendance was not easy due to timing and venues. In the words of one GP:

> We've worked every hour and above God sends and it is very difficult to drop everything for a Social Services conference, it is usually at a place which is difficult to get to... a terrible waste of time.

Predictably, social workers had different views:

> We appreciate the difficulties and it isn't regarded as a criticism but it's just that the GP is a key person here and I'm just wondering whether it is that we are not giving enough notice or the timing isn't right or is it a reluctance to be involved... Child protection really involves putting pieces of a jigsaw together and sometimes we don't know whether the GP knows much about the family... I really regret it when the GP isn't able to come.

These later findings would suggest that perhaps attitudinal issues upon the part of GPs might also play a part in their poor conference attendance.

Parental participation

It should be remembered that parents and carers are now usually invited to attend child protection case conferences, not only to allow them the chance to give their views and opinions but also to hear the concerns that professionals have expressed about their children. The parent with parental responsibility is always invited to attend, even when parents are not living together. In exceptional circumstances, the conference chair may decide to exclude one or both parents if there is a perceived risk of violent behaviour or disruption to the information sharing and decision-making processes.

Child protection case conferences may be intimidating for both parents and professionals. Initially health professionals, especially paediatricians, were ambivalent to the concept of parental attendance at CPCCs. It was argued that professionals would be uncomfortable with parental presence and this could prevent them from expressing perceived criticisms of parents at the meeting (Skeffington 1993). Parents, on the other hand, would be intimidated by being scrutinized by a large number of professionals. While acknowledging these concerns, it is now felt that parental attendance is to be encouraged wherever possible (Hutchinson 1993).

It is essential that parents are adequately prepared prior to the conference. All participants, including parents, should be fully briefed regarding the purpose and process of the conference. All reports submitted by professionals before the conference should be shared with the parents so that they have time to absorb the relevant information. It is understandably difficult for parents to hear negative or critical information for the first time in public. Parents are advised that reports will not be changed if they disagree with the contents; however, they are empowered to give their views during the conference.

Parents are encouraged to invite a friend or family member to accompany them to the conference. Some may choose to bring their legal adviser. It should be remembered that in this context, solicitors may only fulfil the role of an advisor or supporter. They are not entitled to undertake a confrontational or adversarial role more usually associated with the courtroom.

Report writing

Professionals who are invited to a CPCC may be asked to provide a written report outlining their involvement with a child and his/her family, which will be shared with other participants at the conference. GPs will already be aware that personal information about children and their families held by professionals is subject to a legal duty of confidentiality and should not normally be disclosed without the consent of the subject concerned. However the law permits the disclosure of confidential information if it is necessary to safeguard a child or children in the public interest.

It is recognized good practice to seek consent from parents in order to share information that will be disseminated at the CPCC. It is therefore important to discuss with the parents/carers the reasons for sharing such information. Sometimes the GP may have ethical objections to sharing particularly sensitive information with outside agencies. On occasion, parents may object to certain information being made public. In this case, the GP should discuss these areas of difficulty with the CPCC chair or a senior Social Worker.

The following practical points may be of use when compiling a report for a conference: Schedule 1 of the Data Protection Act (1998) requires that information is:

+ shared with others only for the purpose specified (i.e. to facilitate the child protection process)
+ relevant to the specific case and not excessive in length
+ accurate
+ up to date.

The report may include issues such as:

+ attendance rate for appointments at the surgery;
+ seeking appropriate and timely medical care and advice for the child (it is not appropriate to merely submit a computer print out of all attendances at the surgery);
+ notification of frequent attendance at accident and emergency departments;
+ child's growth and development;
+ compliance with medical care;
+ attendance for immunisations and developmental assessments;
+ parenting concerns including drug and alcohol misuse, mental ill health, relationship with the child, parents' expectations of the child;
+ parental ability to understand the reasons for concern and their ability to change.

It is always good practice to record positive aspects of care as well as the areas of concern. This will assist in making an overall assessment of risk to the child.

The way forward

1 Further work is required in order to continue to define the most appropriate ways by which GPs may more effectively participate in the child protection process, especially with respect to attendance at child protection case conferences. Research may be required in order to determine whether newer practices (holding conferences at GPs' surgeries, attending for the first half-hour only, delegation to the practice health visitor) are effective in the representation of a primary care perspective at CPCCs.

2 Following this, there is a need for agreed standards to be developed in this respect between Primary Care Trusts and Area Child Protection Committees.

3 Flexibility and understanding upon the part of both social workers and GPs are required in order to ensure that all relevant information is shared at conferences.

1 Social Services Departments:

♦ need to fully appreciate the GP's role in the provision of health care not only for individual children but also for their families and communities

♦ should give careful consideration to the amount of notice given for conferences, their timing and appropriateness of venue

♦ acknowledge the pressure of GPs' workload and varied commitments

2 GPs, for their part need to:

♦ appreciate the role of social workers in the provision of support for children considered at risk of harm

♦ actively acknowledge the paramountcy principle that places the welfare of children above all other consideration

♦ ensure that a primary care perspective is provided at every child protection case conference either by attending or by providing a report

♦ discuss issues of information sharing with a senior social workers if there are concerns regarding confidentiality.

References

Bannon MJ, Carter YH and Ross E (1999) Perceived barriers to full participation by General Practitioners in the child protection process. *Journal of Interprofessional Care* 13: 239–48.

Birchall E and Hallett C (1995) *Working Together in Child Protection*. London: HMSO.

Bissett A and Hunter D (1992) Child sexual abuse in general practice in North East Scotland. *Health Bulletin* 50: 237–47.

Blom-Cooper L (1987) *A Child in Mind: Protection of Children in a Responsible Society. The Report of the Committee of Inquiry into the Circumstances Surrounding the Death of Kimberly Carlisle*. London: Borough of Greenwich.

Boyter EM, MacLean DW, Zealley HE and Mason K (1983) Non-accidental injury to children: a survey of professional attitudes. *Journal of the Royal College of General Practitioners* 33: 773–5.

Butler-Sloss E (1988) *Report of the Inquiry into Child Abuse in Cleveland*. London: HMSO.

Children Act 1989. London: HMSO.

Data Protection Act (1988). (Chapter 29) London: HMSO.

Gibbons J, Gallagher B and Bell C (1995) *Operating the Child Protection System: A Study of Child Protection Practices in English Local Authorities.* London: HMSO.

Hallett C (1995) Interagency coordination in child protection. London: HMSO.

Hutchison T (1993) Parental participation in case conferences: the case in favour. *Archives of Disease in Childhood* **69**: 455–7.

Lea-Cox C and Hall A (1991) Attendance of general practitioners at child protection case conferences. *British Medical Journal* **302**: 1378–9.

Polnay JC (2000) General practitioners and child protection case conference participation. *Child Abuse Review* **9**: 108–23.

Simpson CM, Simpson RJ, Power KG, Salter A and Williams G (1994) GP's and health visitors' participation in child protection case conferences. *Child Abuse Review* **3**: 211–30.

Skeffington FS (1993) Parental participation in case conferences: the case against *Archives of Disease in Childhood* **69**: 457–8.

Chapter 16

Working together as a team to protect children

Tom Narducci

Child protection: whose responsibility?

In child protection, as in life in general, we sometimes make assumptions. One day we'll learn that this is never a good idea, as they are invariably wrong!

I have worked in child protection since the early 1980s, and like many of my social work colleagues, had assumed that General Practitioners (GPs) and other health professionals had received similar basic training in child protection and the child protection system. Like others, I thought the training provided by the Area Child Protection Committee (ACPC) built upon existing knowledge.

Understandably, given that statement, I shared many of the frustrations highlighted throughout the available research relating to inter-agency working in general, and in particular to the involvement of GPs and other health workers. Apart from health visitors, whom I have always found to be particularly helpful and engaged, I have otherwise been disappointed in what has at times felt like indifference to child protection work within the health sector.

Approximately two years ago, with one of the editors of this book, I implemented a training programme for a number of GP Registrars in the North London. It was only during our discussions that I found my assumptions had been wrong, and some of my frustrations had been unwarranted. I had, previously, wondered at the fact that 'teacher training' did not include a mandatory child protection element. I was amazed when I found that GP training did not either. Given the key role both of these professions have in relation to the early identification of concerns, it seems almost unbelievable that in neither case is child protection seen as a compulsory part of qualification training.

Having said that, I do remain both confused and frustrated, and at times exasperated, at why, twenty six years after the death of Maria Colwell, we are still researching and writing about the need for effective inter-agency working. Numerous inquiries throughout the decades have stressed the need for, and importance of, ongoing communication and cooperation between the agencies. These have not only commented on relationships between GPs and social workers, but to all of the agencies involved.

Rather than repeat the arguments, in this chapter I intend to explore some of the reasons why little progress appears to have been made.

Previous studies have identified a number of issues that have been perceived to obstruct communication and cooperation. These include confidentiality, GPs seeing all family members as patients (thereby restricting their ability to put the interest of the child first), and mistrust of other professionals. Although I will address some of the issues raised by these, I believe focusing on them avoids addressing the real question. In my judgement, the key question with regard to inter-agency child protection working is as follows: whose responsibility is it?

In theory, all agencies share that responsibility. *Working Together to Safeguard Children*,[1] states that:

> Promoting children's well-being and safeguarding them from significant harm depends crucially upon effective information sharing, collaboration and understanding between agencies and professionals.

Both the Scottish Office[2] and the National Assembly for Wales[3] have issued similar guidance for those countries. In each case, there is clear and unambiguous direction for all professionals to share the task of protecting children.

In practice, however, it appears that child protection is seen as the responsibility of Social Service/Social Work Departments, and that other professions merely have a role in supporting them in that task. Perhaps this is the key. Understandably, no one wants to think about child cruelty. It is not a pleasant subject and reminds us of just what we are capable of doing to our own kind. If child protection can be left to others, so much the better, especially when we can legitimize our inaction or limited involvement by identifying it as someone else's responsibility anyway. Our nature is to avoid, when possible, issues that are painful or unpleasant. In child protection, however, by devolving complete responsibility to others, we ignore the adverse consequences for children. And, of course, we can use the failures of those 'others' to justify why we need to be careful of working too closely with them in the future. We know them to be unreliable.

In part, this conflict between stated and perceived roles may be due to the way services for families were split when the National Health Service was first created.[4] The majority of services for families, such as social care and housing, were provided at a local level but health services were delivered at a national level. Furthermore, with the independent and autonomous contractual status of GPs, perhaps it was inevitable that difficulties would arise. However, the question remains: whose responsibility is child protection? Whatever the difficulties, children are still being abused and in too many cases, the system is still failing them.

GPs in particular, and the health services in general, have a key role to play in the protection of children. 'All health professionals, in the NHS, private sector, and other agencies, play an essential part in ensuring that children and families receive the care, support and services they need in order to promote children's health and development.'[5]

Previous research[6] indicates disappointing GP attendance at ACPC training, at child protection case conferences, and also an apparent reluctance to the sharing of information. Many GPs are unaware of the procedures, even at the most basic level of how to undertake child protection register checks. Research has shown that the register was not consulted for 60% of children for whom there were child protection concerns.[7]

Each of the disciplines represented in primary care has contact with children and families on a regular basis. More than any one else, they have the opportunity to identify problems at an early stage, to recognize where and when things are going wrong and to have a real impact. Primary health care staff are likely to be the first to become aware of mental health problems being experienced by parents and carers, of difficulties with drug or alcohol misuse, of domestic violence and of many other factors which may impact negatively on children. Yet experience has shown that in a substantial number of cases, relevant information has not been shared with the other agencies. The opportunities for early intervention have been lost, and a child has not been given the appropriate level of protection.

I would not argue for indiscriminate sharing of confidential medical information. I am also aware of the special relationship that exists between doctor and patient. However, if relevant aspects of a case are not shared with those who may be in a position to help or who have a statutory responsibility to act, this, in my mind, could result in ignoring the needs of the child. According to legislation,[8] the needs of the child should be the primary concern. It must also be remembered that the law permits the disclosure of confidential information necessary to safeguard a child or children in the public interest.[9] Similar guidance issued by the General Medical Council: 'Disclosure of information which may assist in the prevention or detection of abuse, applies both to information about third parties and about children who may be the subject of abuse'.[10]

Framework for the assessment of children in need and their families

The new 'Framework for the Assessment of Children in Need and their Families'[11] confirms the role of GPs and PHCTs in this respect as being ongoing, stating:

> Primary health care team members should know when it is appropriate to refer a child ... to social services for help and support, and how to act on concerns that a child may be at risk of harm through abuse and neglect ... The GP and PHCT will have an important contribution to make to initial and core assessments of children in need. [They] are also well placed to recognise when a parent or other adult has problems which may affect their capacity as a parent or carer or which mean that they pose a risk of harm to a child.

Crucially, the section concludes:

> If they have concerns that an adult's problems or behaviour may be causing, or putting a child at risk of harm, they should follow the procedures set out in *Working Together to Safeguard Children* (1999).

These comments refer not only to the process of referral of concern but also to sharing of information and full integration within the child protection system, which is specifically described within the *Framework* as 'a continuing process and not a single event'. A further point was made in *Messages from Research:*[12] 'the effectiveness (of inter-agency work) tended to decline once child protection plans had been made, with social services left with sole responsibility for implementing the plans'.

So what is it, which really prevents the communication and cooperation referred to at the beginning of this chapter and in almost all research on the subject?

Previous research[13] suggests a number of factors, at different levels. Many GPs still appear unclear as to their role, considering child abuse as an area in which health visitors are better suited. They may also be less confident of making specialized diagnosis, particularly as this is now more likely to be challenged in the courts, and yet the 'designated doctor,' in many areas of the country, remains an underused resource.

There is also the issue of trust between GPs and social workers. Many GPs may have had negative experiences of Social Services in relation to services for the elderly, the mentally ill and/or the disabled. Social Services appear unable to deliver and therefore, there is little point in referring. For their part, social workers may see GPs as remote and unaware of the challenges they face. Arguments of work pressures carry little weight with those struggling to manage large and difficult caseloads and who share the stress of personal accountability. Information they see as necessary and have requested is sometimes refused on the grounds that the GP also has a professional responsibility to the alleged abuser (in cases of abuse within a family). Social workers would argue that they too, have to work with the whole family. As a result, many social workers see little point in trying to involve GPs in child protection work, since they are perceived as being uncooperative and unhelpful – and so the cycle continues.

The concept of dual pathology

All professionals who work in child protection need to recognise that dual pathology exists. In a Department of Health report on Child Abuse Inquiries, undertaken in 1991,[14] dual pathology was recognized in a number of cases. The study states: 'The inquiries are full of instances where, having identified one problem, professionals failed to appreciate another ... The superimposition of one view in pathology over another can (also) take place in time'.

In reaching initial decisions as to the extent of any possible risk to a child, it is imperative to have all the information. The danger of having missing pieces is that, as in a jigsaw, without all the pieces you are unlikely to see the full picture. Instead, you focus on the most obvious bit. However, in so doing you risk missing the true meaning of what is before your eyes. In child protection this can mean for example focusing on one particular incident without having a true picture of the context in which it has occurred. Longer term, the risks are just as real. Few family situations remains unchanged for long and there is an need for continuous sharing of information.

Both GPs and health visitors have raised concerns at what they describe as 'ethical' issues that arise from undertaking a monitoring role in the child protection process. Some perceive this role as a threat to their relationship with the family. It should be remembered that both the British Medical Association and the

Conference of Medical Royal Colleges have consistently highlighted the importance of full participation by doctors within 'all aspects of child protection work'.[15] Furthermore, similar guidance has been produced by the Standing Nursing and Midwifery Advisory Committee.[16]

Child protection is not a single act of intervention. A child is not protected through an investigation and child protection conference alone. The process may begin with those elements – however, that is only the beginning. Each of the professionals involved will have an ongoing role, of which the child and family should be aware. Child protection work requires time and commitment. There are already many GPs, other health staff and social workers in the field working closely together, in line with recommended best practice. Unfortunately, there are many others who appear locked within those arguments which have been well rehearsed throughout the years. This is where change has yet to begin.

The way forward

So how can we move that onward? What steps need to happen which will reduce the isolation, break down barriers and prevent someone sitting down in twenty six years from now to write a chapter on the need to work together as a team in order to best protect children?

Enhanced communication

The pressures on our time restrict our ability to communicate effectively with each other, and without that level of communication, appropriate change is impossible. When serious cases of abuse or the death of a child occur, communication is not usually a significant problem. It is with the 'day-to-day' work that we fail. This is especially the case when it seems reasonable to delegate child protection issues to the health visitor, or to the social worker, or to anyone else. In a similar fashion, it is perhaps easier for social workers to ignore the GP's potential contribution to this process. Rather Social Services should persevere with requests for information, explore ways of increasing the GP's involvement, and arrange child protection case conferences at suitable times and accessible venues.

PCTs

I believe that the creation of Primary Care Trusts (PCTs) presents us with an opportunity for progress. The requirement for all districts to develop Children's Services Plans that actively involve PCTs should be seen as a first step in ensuring common ownership of the local system for protecting children. Child protection is best seen as part of a continuum of services for children and not as some isolated service provided by one agency, with help from the others. GPs will, in future, be well placed to argue the need for greater coordination of local health care services, part of which must be focused on the protection of children from abuse, and the ability of services to respond to it.

Enhancement of community child health

Child Health in the Community[17] has already identified many good practices that should be further developed at a local level. *Childhood Matters*[18] also recognized the role of GPs and health visitors as being central to the overall well-being of children, including in their protection from abuse. (PCTs provide at least part of a structure in which this can begin to happen.) This document made a number of recommendations referring to primary care and to others within health, and, in particular, mental health services. Research into links between adult mental health services and child protection have consistently identified difficulties and recommended closer communication and cooperation if future tragedies are to be prevented. For example, Falkov[19] found evidence of psychiatric illness in the parent/carer in one third of the one hundred Part Eight Case Reviews studied.

More joined-up working and thinking

Links need to be established across what is currently perceived as distinct, separate services for adults and children. There is an urgent need to address communication within disciplines and across them. In the field of mental health, hospital and community health professionals need to liaise more closely and to discuss any possible impact on children of an adult's illness. That information then needs to be shared with social workers in order that appropriate plans for support can be put into place.

These will not be easy tasks to accomplish. This will require the development of trust and must begin with the recognition that

> Each system operates within their own world of ethical issues and unique vocabulary. The particular meaning of concepts . . . is specific to each organisation. In order to work together, common ways of seeing the world must be found by each agency.[20]

Children with disabilities

We must not overlook additional issues that exist with respect to safeguarding children with disabilities. 'The available UK evidence . . . suggest that disabled children are at increased risk of abuse, and . . . multiple disabilities appears to increase the risk.'[21]

The new *Framework for Assessment* referred to earlier requires a significant commitment from health staff, especially with respect to advising social services of children with additional needs resulting from disability. But even without these guidelines, the needs of a child with a disability (and his family) are self-evident.

Children with disabilities require the services of both health and social services staff. We need to give the same consideration to the improvements we can bring to the lives of 'young carers' and to those children 'looked after' by local authorities, through our working together more effectively. The Government, in its 'Response to the Children's Safeguard Review',[22] has provided a range of recommendations relating to the role of the health services in general, and GPs in particular, in relation to the needs of children in care.

The need for training

I feel that many of the challenges identified in this chapter can be resolved by means of effective training. However, we all need to accept that protecting children from abuse is a shared responsibility. We cannot move on to look at how best that might happen, without the fundamental question posed earlier – 'Whose responsibility is child protection?' first being answered as, 'All of ours.'

It also relies on how we define 'training' and what we see as its purpose (see Chapter 5). If training is only considered as developing the skills and knowledge necessary to carry out specific task or duties then it is unlikely to have the necessary impact. True, GPs, health visitors and other health staff do need to have a basic awareness of child protection. They need to understand what child abuse is, the forms it takes and some of the causes, as well as its impact and how to recognize it. These are the basics that can and should be gained through input during their qualification training.

If, however, we consider the concept of learning, rather than training, many more opportunities become possible. Inter-agency training should not, as happens in some parts of the country, focus on definitions and signs and indicators. Instead, it should be used as a way of enabling the various professions to learn from, and equally importantly about, each other. Inter-agency training 'can be a highly effective way of promoting a common and shared understanding of the respective roles and responsibilities of different professionals and can contribute to effective working relationships'. 'Training should create an ethos which values working collaboratively . . . ' and 'should focus on the way in which those engaged in child welfare work with others to meet the needs of children'.[23] It is possible, but it does require the will of those developing the training and, most especially, of those at whom it is aimed. GPs, for the most part, are not able to cancel or rearrange surgeries. Teachers cannot leave classrooms unattended and schools do not have the funds for locum teachers. Social workers cannot always control their own diaries. There are dozens of reasons why training has failed to bring us together, but not one of them cannot be overcome if we tried, if we were simply more imaginative, creative and flexible.

If we recognized our shared responsibility and the simple fact that without our working together children will continue to suffer, we could overcome these and every other block to effectively protecting children which has been identified.

We can do it and we should do it. The question is will we do it?

References

1   Department of Health, Home Office, Department for Education and Employment (1999) *Working Together to Safeguard Children*, section 1.10. The Stationery Office, London: HMSO.

2   The Scottish Office (1998) *Protecting Children A Shared Responsibility*. The Stationery Office, Edinburgh: HMSO.

3   The National Assembly for Wales (1999) *Working Together to Safeguard Children*. The Stationery Office, London: HMSO.

4   Community Care, Issue 1156, Another Fine Mess, 30 January 1997, article, Anna Coote-Author, page 16. Reed Business Information, Sutton, Surrey.

5   Department of Health, Home Office, Department for Education and Employment (1999) *Working Together to Safeguard Children*, section 3.18. London: HMSO.

6   University of Portsmouth (1999) *The Role of Health Professionals in the Child Protection Process*, Report No. 41, section 1.3. Univ. of Portsmouth Social Services Research and Information Unit.

7   Department of Health, Home Office, Department for Education and Employment (2000) *Framework for the Assessment of Children in Need and their Families*. London: HMSO.

8   The Children Act (1991) The Children (Scotland) Act 1995, The Children (Northern Ireland) Order 1995. London: HMSO.

9   Department of Health, Home Office, Department for Education and Employment (1999) *Working Together to Safeguard Children*, section 7.32. London: HMSO.

10 Department of Health, Home Office, Department for Education and Employment (1999) *Working Together to Safeguard Children*, section 7.43. London: HMSO.

11 Department of Health, Home Office, Department for Education and Employment (2000) *Framework for the Assessment of Children in Need and their Families*, sections 5.22 and 5.23. London: HMSO.

12 Department of Health (1995) *Child Protection – Messages from Research*. London: HMSO.

13 University of Portsmouth (1999) *The Role of Health Professionals in the Child Protection Process*, Report No. 41, section 1.3. Univ. of Portsmouth Social Services Research and Information Unit.

14 Department of Health (1991) *Child Abuse A Study of Inquiry Reports 1980–1989*, section 4.2. London: HMSO.

15 Department of Health, British Medical Association, Conference of Medical Royal Colleges, Child Protection: Medical Responsibilities, section 1.1. London: HMSO (Undated).

16 Department of Health (1997) *Guidance for Senior Nurses, Health Visitors and Midwives and their Managers*. London: HMSO.

17 NHS Executive (1996) *Child Health in the Community*. London: HMSO.

18 NSPCC (1997) *Childhood Matters The Report of the National Commission of Inquiry into the Prevention of Child Abuse*. London: HMSO.

19 Falkov A (1996) *Department of Health, Study of Working Together 'Part 8' Reports, Fatal Child Abuse and Parental Psychiatric Disorder*. London: HMSO.

20 Tye C and Precey G (1999) Building bridges: the interface between adult mental health and child protection. *Child Abuse Review* 8: 164–71. Chichester: Wiley.

21 Department of Health, Home Office, Department for Education and Employment (1999) *Working Together to Safeguard Children*, section 6.27. London: HMSO.

22 The Government's Response to the Children's Safeguards Review (1998). London: HMSO.

23 Department of Health, Home Office, Department for Education and Employment (1999) *Working Together to Safeguard Children*, sections 9.2–9.4. London: HMSO.

Chapter 17

The health needs of looked after children and the role of the primary care team

Mary Mather

Introduction – small things matter

A young care leaver, speaking at a seminar, was asked by a member of the audience what had made him a 'success' despite the difficulties he had experienced growing up in care. He cited as an example someone who had listened to him, a doctor who had seen him as a child. He asked the doctor 'Do you sometimes give people drugs just to keep them quiet?' The doctor replied that he didn't, but that it was an interesting question and he should keep on asking questions. This single remark by a doctor had made him feel valued, had given him positive encouragement and made him feel that he could make a contribution to society.

All general practitioners, often without appreciating the significance, will encounter looked after children during their working lives. Interested and compassionate general practitioners can make a real difference in the lives of young people in the care system.

Why is the health of looked after children included in a book on child protection?

Of the children involved in the child protection process, 96% remain at home with their parents, and the vast majority of those who are removed swiftly return home (Department of Health 1995). However every year a small number of children will be permanently removed from the care of their parents and become the responsibility of the state for part or all of their childhood. Other children will enter the care system because their birth parents cannot care for them, cope with their behaviour, or because their families have abandoned them.

The children for whom substitute parents are now sought are likely to have complex physical, developmental, emotional and educational needs, secondary to the damage caused by inadequate parenting, abuse and neglect. An unpublished study in

Wales (Payne 2000) showed that 71% of looked after children had been on child protection registers within the last 12 months.

The medical skill and experience needed to support the substitute care of children has changed dramatically during the course of this century. Adoption and fostering are increasingly seen as a solution to the problems posed for society by children whose parents are unable, unwilling or judged by the legal system as unfit to care for them.

This group of children and young people, who have not had a high priority in strategic planning, are currently the subjects of two large Government investment programmes: 'Quality Protects' in England and 'Children First' in Wales.

As far as their health is concerned, research has been very limited. This is despite increasing evidence that health care, as it is presently organized, fails most of these children while the health services offered to them are undervalued and often rejected.

Who are looked after children?

Under the Children Act 1989, a child is 'looked after' by a local authority if he or she is placed in their care by a court (under a care order) or provided with accommodation by social services for more than 24 hours.

Figure 17.1 illustrates the recent trends in the numbers of looked after children in England. Following a fall from a peak of almost 100,000 in the early 1980s to 49,000 in 1994, the population is slowly rising again. The numbers of looked after children have increased by 13% between 1994 and 1999 to reach 55,300.

The majority of looked after children (65%) are in foster homes. Less than 9% are in residential community homes. Very few children will move into the security of an

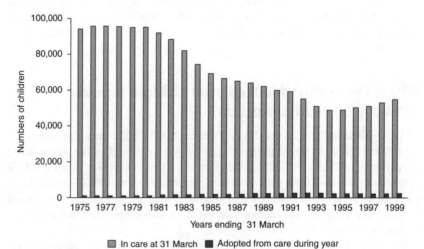

Figure 17.1 Numbers of children looked after and adopted 1975–1999.
Source: DH analysis for PIU team, April 2000.

Age	1994 %	1999 %
Under 1	3	4
1–4	13	17
5–9	21	23
10–15	43	40
16 plus	20	16

Figure 17.2 Change in age profile of looked after children.
Source: DH analysis for PIU team, April 2000.

adoptive family. In 1998/9 only 2,200 children were adopted from the care system, a rate of 4%.

Figure 17.2 shows the way in which the age profile of looked after children has changed between 1994 and 1999. The population is becoming younger; with a 49% increase in the number under one and a 45% increase in children between one and four. More than half the population of looked after children (56%) are over the age of 10 (Prime Minister's Review of Adaption 2000). This group will include older children entering the care system for the first time and those who have grown up in care.

The population is split between those children who move rapidly in and out of substitute care and those who stay longer. The majority of these children spend only brief periods of time in the care system, before returning home. However, a significant number will remain in the system on a long-term basis. About 40% of all children looked after on 31 March 1999 had been in care for 3 years or more. The longer a child remains in care the less the chance of successfully returning home. (Prime Minister's Review of Adoption 2000).

Children with disabilities and learning difficulties are over-represented in this population of children (Department of Health 1998). Many have suffered emotional, sexual or physical abuse. Some are looked after because of risks posed by their parent's lifestyle, e.g. foetal exposure to effects of alcohol or drugs (Macnamara *et al.* 1995). Others may be born to parents suffering from genetically inherited conditions such as schizophrenia.

Children from ethnic minority backgrounds suffer particular discrimination. For many years national statistics were not kept on ethnicity, and there is little research on the health of these children before or after they enter the care system and the effects of social discrimination and poverty on their health status.

Many children will have experienced interrupted or damaged attachment patterns in their early lives and will have continuing attachment difficulties in care causing a range behavioural difficulties. (Fahlberg 1994; Jewitt 1995).

Some children will have multiple difficulties causing complex medical and developmental problems. All will suffer stigma, the disruption of relationships, interrupted education, confusion, bewilderment and loss.

The state as a corporate parent

Children who cannot be brought up by their birth parents have the same rights as other children. The House of Commons (1998) Report on the Health of Children Looked after by Local Authorities was a damning indictment of the failure of the State as a corporate parent.

In 1996, 50–75% of those leaving care had no academic qualifications, compared with 6% of the general population; 12–19% of those leaving care continued in further education compared with 66% the general population; 26% of adolescents aged 14–16 years and 33% of those residential care were not in education.

Of looked after adolescents, 66% had mental health problems compared with 15% of the population; 23% had a major depressive illness compared with 4% of the population and 14% of looked-after girls became pregnant in care or within a year of leaving. A national drug and alcohol survey found that 44% of substance abusers had been in care: 50% of young people living rough and 40% of the prison population are care leavers.

These poor outcomes occur even though it is a statutory requirement that all children in the care system should have regular medical examinations. A registered medical practitioner should carry out these examinations within one month of entry into the care system (HMSO 1991b). Subsequently, the examination must be repeated every six months if the child is under two years and annually for those over two years. No other group of children in the population is subject to this statutory requirement (HMSO 1991b, 1997a).

How relevant is the statutory medical examination in practice?

There are only two published studies evaluating a statutory obligation as a mechanism to protect health. The first, a survey carried out Mather et al. (1997) in south-east London, examined 219 medical reports on 194 children looked after over a period of two years between 1994–96. Eighty-seven of these children were adolescents; 10% of the children had no registered general practitioner; 27.5% had an abnormal birth history; 38% of their mothers had chronic ill health; 48% were either educationally statemented or had significant school problems; 67% had been referred to child guidance or had major behavioural problems. Perhaps most significantly the number of medicals carried out represented an uptake of only 25%.

The second study was conducted by Butler and Payne (1997) in Cardiff audited the medical records of a randomly chosen group of 199 looked after children. The uptake was identical at 25%. There was no difference in coverage between children placed with their parents, in foster care or in residential care – 50% had not even been invited for a medical examination.

Why should a system with so many legal safeguards and to which a large amount of health service resource is devoted produce such an unsatisfactory situation?

Why are health outcomes so poor?

Before being looked after, health is often neglected due to poverty, poor diet or poor housing. Many children will have missed routine child health surveillance, immunization, hospital appointments, vision, hearing and dental checks. Absence or exclusion from school produces educational failure, which impacts on health. Particularly important is the damage to the child's self-esteem caused by inconsistent or bad parenting.

Why are there no conspicuous improvements in health once a child is in the care system? Here again, the record is depressing. Many children experience frequent changes of social worker, foster carer and of school. Poor record keeping and the delayed transmission of health records compound this situation. No previous medical records encourages over-reliance on isolated, uncoordinated medical examinations. Many children are not registered with general practitioners. Poor communication between health and social services leads to confusion about who is responsible for action. There can be difficulties in obtaining consent or delegated consent for medical treatment.

Most parents see it as their responsibility to carry out the day to day monitoring of their child's health. In the care system it is rare that an equivalent responsibility is undertaken. Health and social services professionals used to acute short-term interventions at a time of crisis are ill equipped to carry the responsibility for an individual child's health over a long period of time (Parker et al. 1991).

Advantaged children have a resilience that enables them to cope better with adversity than deprived children. Children deprived of parents are often driven into a cycle of ill health that contributes to their ultimate social exclusion and unhappiness, and are often wary or rejecting of health contacts. If children in the care system are to achieve the same state of health as children brought up within their own family, then a radical change in the delivery of their health care is needed.

What young people said

Young people in care rightly have views about the services they need, and it is essential to consider them if substantial progress is to be made in improving their health outcomes. A survey in 1997 (Mather et al. 1997) sought the views of young people in the care system. Their demands were modest and yet spoke volumes about the system's failure to address their needs.

Young people resented the physical examination. As one young woman said 'Having to take your clothes off for a strange doctor, when you don't feel ill is yet one more abuse'. Having medical examinations when they were not ill made little sense. Few knew they had any choice and those who did frequently refused to attend. All had experienced a lack of opportunity to discuss basic health care, but medicals were not seen as an opportunity to redress this problem. A visit to a doctor was about getting medicine because they were ill. Asking for advice on general or sexual health was not on their agenda.

Confidentiality was of serious concern. Many did not trust the doctor to keep what they said confidential. The fact that medical reports were sent to their social workers emerged as a major deterrent to seeking medical care, because intimate details about their health were discussed and disseminated as if everyone had a right to know. Some expressed the view that meetings about their health were conducted as if they were not present. Health professionals were sometimes perceived to be insensitive about the difficulties of living in the care system.

The young people talked overwhelmingly about depression, isolation and the lack of a trusted adult in whom to confide whilst struggling with unresolved issues of loss, bereavement and separation. Against this background it was difficult to take a pro-active approach to health. As one young woman (aged 14) said, 'If you feel so bad about yourself and what has happened to you, what does it matter if you take risks with your health anyway?'

The young people lacked basic health information. They wanted information about skin and hair care, diet, eating disorders, exercise, contraception and drugs but found it difficult to access appropriate advice, getting it mainly from television, magazines and from each other. There was a real lack of opportunity for discussion about risk-taking behaviour, and often those who cared for them were too embarrassed to help them think through the issues.

For those in residential care, where there was a lot of peer pressure not to go to bed early, rest and sleep were of particular concern. For others, bedtime had very trau-matic associations but few were able to talk to anybody about these feelings. Several young people referred to being surrounded by adults who smoked. Some had not smoked prior to being looked after, but had started because of peer pressure and living in an environment where smoking was the norm.

The way forward: health assessments not medical examinations

A radically new approach is needed, concentrating on holistic health care and empha-sizing health, not illness. Rather than a medical examination, children in care should be offered an annual opportunity to meet with a health professional to discuss issues of concern.

In the future nurses may be the professionals who befriend vulnerable children, particularly if the annual health assessment can be carried out at school, or as part of routine child health surveillance within primary care. A doctor or nurse who thinks in terms of a health assessment as a joint exercise with their young patients, and who encourages them to talk about his or her own health will be most successful. The child's contact with the primary health care team should be tolerant, understanding and non-stigmatizing.

In most cases general practitioners will remain responsible for the annual health assessments. Superficially this seems to be a simple medical task. However, for a child in perfect health, singled out in the family or classroom for a visit to the doctor, it can seem stigmatizing and pointless. The doctor will have to explain and sometimes justify what the child may see as unnecessary. Both foster carer and child will need support and sensitive handling by the general practitioner.

Although physical examination is seen as important by social workers, very few doctors are convinced of the efficacy or usefulness of it as a routine annual event in healthy children. Young people themselves are often very fearful of physical examina-tion, which can sometimes bring back painful memories of past abuse. Examining doctors must recognize that these feelings are often justified by the children's experience of care system bureaucracy and of abuse and its consequences. An initial statement of 'you don't have to be examined if you don't want to' will not only help the young patient to relax, but will also, paradoxically, increase the chance of a later successful examination.

Older children, wherever possible, should be able to choose the doctor or nurse who carries out a health assessment. It can also be very reassuring if that professional is of the same ethnic group or gender as the child.

Even if the child is not physically examined a health assessment is a useful opportunity for the general practitioner to meet the child, to explain the services offered in the practice, perhaps offer a nurse assessment and to discuss preventative health care. Vision, hearing, immunization, sexual health, smoking and dental care are all important health issues. Like any good parent it is better to address these problems early in the child's life than to tackle them in adolescence or when the young person leaves care.

Adults brought up in care often have no knowledge about their own personal medical history or of significant medical problems in their birth family. The general practitioner might be in a position to give some of this information to the child by sharing his records with the patient.

All children and young people in public care should have:

◆ A National Health Service number

◆ A named general practitioner

◆ A named dentist

◆ An accurate record of medical treatment, illness, operations and hospital visits

◆ An accurate record of dental care and treatment

◆ An accurate immunization record with dates

◆ Regular vision and hearing checks

◆ An individual health plan

The child's informed consent, actively sought and recorded, is paramount. The child's consent to the release of confidential medical information should also be actively sought at each episode of health care.

Looked after children frequently come from backgrounds of abuse and neglect. The trauma of their early years has long-lasting effects on physical and mental health, development, education, and behaviour. The assessment of these often damaged children must be done by general practitioners experienced in child and adolescent health who are able to complete a holistic assessment. A Consultant Community Paediatrician should see all children with particularly complex problems.

Adolescents

Adolescents make up a high proportion of looked after children (Sinclair *et al.* 1995; Cleaver 1996) and are the group most likely to refuse a medical. Some will make this refusal very clear. They should be encouraged to take part in a similar process of health assessment with the reassurance that the assessment will not be repeated unless there is a good reason. It is good practice to offer adolescents copies of all health reports written about them.

Teenagers and young people must be treated with great sensitivity and their rights recognized. Any child or young person deemed to be capable of understanding the reasons for an examination has the legal right of consent and hence to refuse consent. Under the Gillick ruling it is a matter for the doctor's professional judgement whether a child under sixteen is sufficiently responsible to make decisions about their own health (Gillick 1985).

Adolescents, judged to be Gillick competent, are entitled to seek medical treatment without the consent of their foster carer or social worker. Unsupported adolescents are at risk of early sexual activity, with the consequences of unplanned pregnancy and sexually transmitted disease. They have a right to access family planning, emergency contraception, and other sexual health services without the knowledge or consent of the adults responsible for them. Work with adolescents suggests that they will only access these services if they have absolute confidence in the health care professionals treating them and that confidentiality will be maintained.

Foster-carers

Foster-carers are in a unique position to observe children in their care and are nearly always very effective advocates for them. It is the foster carer's task to ensure that all looked after children receive appropriate health care. They should feel able to seek advice from their general practitioner whenever they have concerns about a child.

All foster carers should have written information from Social Services, which they can share with their general practitioner, indicating when they are allowed to give consent for medical treatment. This is especially important for preventative services such as dental checks, immunizations and routine child health surveillance. Any action or recommendation following a medical should clearly identify who is responsible for that action and within what time scale the actions will be carried out.

Failure of the child's birth parent to give consent for medical treatment should not be allowed to override a child's need for health care. The reassuring advice of the general practitioner can be very important in this case. Social workers are not medically trained and are often very hesitant about the responsibility of consenting to such procedures as immunization.

Smoking by substitute carers is a controversial area. In the past doctors have attracted negative publicity by refusing to let smokers care for children on health grounds. However, foster carers who smoke need to prevent the exposure of children and young people to passive cigarette smoke. It is particularly tragic when previously non-smoking young people come into the care system and become smokers themselves as a result of the example of their carers.

It is good practice to offer all residential staff and foster carers immunization against Hepatitis B.

Looked after children, records and registration

No looked after child should be registered as a temporary resident with a general practitioner. Full registration is essential. Whilst all health staff recognize that only full registration gives a child the opportunity to build a lasting confidential relationship with their doctor, this is not widely known within social services or by foster carers. General practitioners will need to provide continuity of care, ensure they receive the child's previous NHS records and give the child the opportunity for preventative healthcare within the primary care team. Full registration is therefore essential.

For a child who is brought up within its birth family, there is little need to depend on accurate medical record keeping. Most parents have an intimate knowledge of their own child's health and development. For children separated from their families, all too frequently the story is one of loss or delay in the transfer of medical records, disrupted medical histories and inadequate record keeping. The continuity of medical records is vital for children. For looked after children, who often have less than optimal health, failures in medical record keeping can have very serious consequences.

General practitioners, who are responsible for a child's healthcare, must ensure that they have access to key health information held by the local authority about a child. They should request this information from the social worker before seeing a child or before the child joins their list. Doctors should not undertake health care in the absence of this information. Sadly, it remains too common for a child to present at the surgery with no records and a foster carer who has only known a child for a few weeks. Consultations done in these circumstances, unless a child is acutely ill, are dangerous, unhelpful to the child and a waste of health service resources.

The health assessment of substitute carers

The primary health care team has an important role to play in the assessment of the health of substitute carers. Most general practitioners will have completed the British Agencies for Adoption and Fostering (BAAF) Adult 1 form, which is normally required for all adults seeking to provide substitute care for children.

General practitioners should be aware that this exercise is focused on the child rather than on the adult, although it is understandable that doctors are sometimes anxious not to jeopardize a patient's chances of caring for a child. Medical information is by no means the only criteria on which social service's decisions are made. Fostered and adopted children bring many challenges. They need parents who are robust both mentally and physically and sensitive to a child's background and birth family. The ability to parent is more important than perfect health.

A doctor needs to make an honest assessment of a patient's ability to care for a child. It is important that this is a factual, documented account, which the patient can see. These forms often provide the general practitioner with a genuine conflict of loyalty. There is a wide variation between general practitioners in the information that they believe to be relevant. The general practitioner who writes, 'slightly depressed' or 'drinks more than normal' or 'marital problems' may be genuinely trying to be helpful to the medical adviser whilst struggling to maintain the patient's confidentiality and trust.

Honesty with patients is important and is the only way to prevent painful situations developing in the future. It is good practice to discuss any concerns honestly with the applicant. General practitioners should remember that adults whose application is turned down by an agency have the right to request a reconsideration of their application. They also have a right to know on what grounds they were rejected as substitute carers. Unless general practitioners are honest with patients from the beginning, an extremely angry patient could face them several months later demanding to know what had been said about them behind their back.

Confidential telephone calls to the local authority medical adviser about a specific patient without the patient's knowledge should be avoided whenever possible. The medical adviser is then placed in the impossible situation of not knowing to whom this confidential information should be revealed, while at the same time trying to act in the best interests of the child.

Children can arrive in substitute families, whether foster or adoptive, by various routes. Substitute families have been trained to expect and deal with the difficulties of these children. Most would-be foster-carers are competent, skilled and compassionate people who have been selected by their agencies for their potential as substitute parents. When difficulties arise they may be reluctant to return to their agencies for fear that they are seen to be failures. No such inhibitions may exist regarding the doctor's surgery, and they may initially confide their difficulties to their general practitioners. Placements in difficulties require support rather than the removal of the child. The general practitioner's traditional role as the family's advocate will be invaluable at times like this, supporting the foster-carer and child until appropriate help is provided.

Birth parents

The general practitioner's first encounter with substitute care may be with birth parents that have had a child removed from their care. Parting with a child has a life-long profound emotional impact. Even when the physical separation has taken place years previously, isolated events at a later date can reactivate feelings of loss. General practitioners need to offer appropriate non-judgemental support.

Birth mothers (Howe et al. 1992) and sometimes fathers retain this sense of loss throughout their lives. Unresolved grief can impair relationships with partners or subsequent children. Doctors unfamiliar with the implications of substitute care may not recognize the effects of this early trauma, yet it can underline a whole range of chronic psychosomatic illnesses and may lead to the inappropriate use of primary care. Some doctors will enter 'child adopted' on a patient's record without realizing the significance. A few minutes spent examining what this means to this patient will not only strengthen the doctor–patient relationship but will also lead to the sharing of valuable information.

Abuse in substitute care

It is tempting to assume that children who are in foster care are safe from further abuse. Abuse however continues in both residential and foster homes. For those placed on child protection registers as of 31 March 1999, 25% were looked after (Department of Health 1999). The whole question of abuse in substitute care has received renewed attention with the publication of Sir William Utting's Report on the safeguards for children living away from home (Department of Health and the Welsh Office 1997) and the Waterhouse North Wales public enquiry into residential homes in Wales (Department of Health 2000).

Vulnerability, isolation, the lack of an independent complaints procedure and reluctance on the part of adults to listen to children may mean that further abuse goes unrecognized. Looked after children can be emotionally or physically abused by over-burdened foster carers who are expected to manage behaviourally disturbed children with little support. Other children in the same placement can also abuse children. A study in Leeds (Hobbs *et al.* 1999) found 41% incidents of abuse in substitute care involved the foster parents, 23% took place during contact with birth parents and 20% involved another child, either a sibling, another foster child or the children of the foster family.

The general practitioner needs to remain alert to the possibility that looked after children will suffer further abuse. Deterioration in behaviour or persistent running away from the placement may be important warning signs. Despite the importance of confidentiality, any disclosure of abuse made by a looked after child within the context of health care must be reported to the social services under the child protection procedures. (Department of Health 1991).

The GP as commissioner – Primary Care Trusts

After the 1997 general election there was a fundamental change in the direction and organization of the National Health Service, which increasingly will become primary care led. The medical support for adoption and fostering services has traditionally been 'invisible' to general practitioners. It is important that commissioning general practitioners, along with their colleagues from social services, ensure that these children have health services which will meet their needs.

These children will need specialized secondary and tertiary paediatric care for many years. General practitioners will need to work proactively with both community paediatricians and child psychiatrists to commission services for looked after children. Particular attention should be given to the high incidence of behaviour problems and the lack of resources for effective mental health interventions.

The future aspirations for the services for looked after children must be a determination to reverse the inequalities in health, which exist between children cared for by the State and those brought up by their families. This will involve moving from medical examinations to health care, using a mix of health care professionals to meet their needs and a closer monitoring of both the quality of service provide and the health outcomes for the children.

Acknowledgement

This chapter is based on material previously published as *Doctors for Children in Public Care, Advocating, Promoting and Protecting Health* by Mather and Batty published by British Agencies for Adoption and Fostering (BAAF) 200 Union Street, London SE1 0LX. The material is reproduced by kind permission of the publishers.

References

Butler I and Payne H (1997) The health of children looked after by the local authority. *Adoption and Fostering* 21(2): 28–35.

Cleaver H (1996) *Focus on Teenagers*. London: HMSO.

Department of Health, Home Office and Department of Education and Science (1991) *Working Together Under the Children Act (1989): A Guide to Interagency Co-operation for the Protection of Children*. London: HMSO.

Department of Health (1995) *Child Protection Messages from Research*. London: HMSO.

Department of Health and the Welsh Office (1997) *People like us: The Report of the Review of the Safeguards for Children living away from Home, Sir William Utting*. HMSO: London.

Department of Health (1998) *Quality Protects: Transforming Children's Services: Objectives for Social Services*. London: HMSO.

Department of Health (1999) *Statistical Bulletin: Government Statistical Service*. London

Department of Health (2000) *Lost in Care – Report of the Tribunal of Inquiry into the Abuse of Children in Care in the Former County Council Areas of Gwynedd and Clwyd since 1974*. London: HMSO.

Fahlberg V (1994) *A Child's Journey Through Placement*. London: British Agencies for Adoption and Fostering.

Gillick (1985) Gillick v Norfolk (Wisbech Division) Area Health Authority and Department of Health and Social Security (Statutory Instrument No. 3allER402).

Hobbs G, Hobbs J and Wynne J (1999) Abuse of children in foster and residential care. *Child Abuse and Neglect* 23(12): 1239–52.

HMSO (1991b) *The Approval of Households: Placement of Children Regulations 1991*. London: HMSO.

HMSO (1997a) *The Adoption Agencies and Children (Arrangements for Placements and Reviews) (Miscellaneous Amendments) Regulations 1997*. London: HMSO.

House of Commons (1998) *The Health of Children Looked after by Local Authorities: Report of the Department of Health Select Committee*. London: HMSO.

Howe D, Sawbridge P and Hingings D (1992) *Half a Million Women: Mothers who Lose their Children*. London: Penguin.

Jewitt C (1995) *Helping Children Cope With Separation And Loss*. London: British Agencies for Adoption and Fostering.

Macnamara J, Bullock A and Grimes E (1995) *Bruised before Birth*. London: British Agencies for Adoption and Fostering.

Mather M, Humphrey J and Robson J (1997) The statutory medical and health needs of looked after children. *Adoption and Fostering* 21(2): 35–40.

Parker R, Ward H, Jackson S, Aldgate J and Wedge P (eds) (1991) *Assessing Outcomes in Child Care*. London: HMSO.

Payne H (2000) Senior lecturer, University of Wales, College of Medicine, Personal communication.

Prime Minister's Review of Adoption (2000) A Consultation Document, Performance and Innovation Unit Cabinet Office. London, July 2000.

Rowe J and Lambert L (1975) *Children Who Wait, British Agencies for Adoption and Fostering.* London.

Saunders L and Broad B (1997) *The Health of Young People Leaving Care.* Centre for Social Action, Leicester: de Montford University.

Sinclair R, Garnett L and Berridge D (1995) *Social Work and Assessment with Adolescents.* London: National Childrens Bureau.

Chapter 18

Child protection and primary care organizations (PCOs)

Ruth Bastable

Introduction

Rita, in Willy Russell's *Educating Rita* (1996) was asked how she would present Ibsen's very long and complex play *Peer Gynt*. Her essay in its entirety was, 'Do it on the radio'. Asked how I would put child protection on the Primary Care Organization (PCO) agenda, I would reply in a similar vein – 'Put it in the HImP' (Health Improvement Programme). But like Rita, I have discovered there's more to it than that. This chapter describes the latest reorganization of the NHS in England, with particular emphasis on the changes affecting primary care. This reorganization is then related to how change in primary care, and particularly change in general practice, can be brought about. Finally, the potential for change is related specifically to child protection issues. Most of the comments, particularly with respect to accountability and governance, apply to Scotland and Wales as well as England. The chapter will have interest for all those working in primary care, but will be especially relevant for those wishing to see change in how child protection issues are managed within the general practice setting. PCOs are very new, they went 'live' on 1 April 1999 and already some Primary Care Groups (PCGs) have made the transition to Primary Care Trusts (PCTs) (Audit Commission 2000). All PCGs remaining have to work towards trust status (Department of Health 2000) so sampling this chapter will be a bit like sampling a half-cooked cake. We are in a period of significant change, not to say turbulence, within the NHS, and no one is quite sure how it will all turn out.

The new NHS

Primary Care Organizations (PCOs) made their first appearance as Primary Care Groups (PCGs) in the White Paper *The New NHS: Modern, Dependable* (Department of Health 1997) which set out the government's proposals for the reorganization of the NHS. The lynchpin of this was to change the way the NHS was run by replacing the internal market of fundholding with a system of 'integrated care, based on part-nership and driven by performance'. With commissioning of care comes accountability for that care, and a concern for quality and financial propriety which would belong to both clinical and non-clinical staff, representing an alignment of clinical as well as financial responsibility.

From 1 April 1999, every general practice and every general practitioner in England has had to belong to a PCO. Unlike fundholding, which involved about 60% of English GPs, (Audit Commission 2000) there is no opt-out clause and unlike fund-holding, where the emphasis was on a market economy and competition within primary care, the emphasis of the latest reorganization is on quality, collaboration and cooperation. At a minimum (level 1) and operating as a subcommittee of the Health Authority, a PCG must support and advise the Health Authority on commissioning of services for the local population the PCG represents (NHS Executive 1998). At level 2, the PCG assumes responsibility for commissioning services for the local community and managing health care budgets, but again as a Health Authority subcommittee. PCOs at level 3 and 4, known as Primary Care Trusts (PCTs), are free standing bodies independent of the Health Authority, although they remain account-able to it. Trusts at level 3 will commission *and provide* health care, those at level 4 will commission health care *and* community services *and provide* those services. PCTs at level 4 will amalgamate with local community trusts and therefore become the employer for all relevant community staff (such as health visitors and district nurses). It is also envisaged that PCTs, as Care Trusts (Department of Health 2000), will commission some aspects of social care related to health.

The precise form of the PCGs and the rate at which they will proceed to trust status is flexible, and reflects local circumstances, but PCGs are obliged to move to trust status by 2004 (Department of Health 2000).

The position in Scotland and Wales is slightly different. Membership of Scotland's Local Health Care Cooperatives (LHCCs) is voluntary, but a majority of Scottish practices belong (SHOW 2000). LHCCs do not hold budgets or commission services, but have other elements of responsibility akin to PCGs; notably they have to make arrangements for clinical governance.

Local Health Groups (LHGs) in Wales are constituted as sub committees of the Health Authority. GPs are obliged to belong. LHGs have advisory *and* commissioning responsibilities, and again have to make arrangements for clinical governance (NHS Wales 1998).

What PCOs do

PCOs have three major areas of responsibility. These are: commissioning services, developing services, and improving the health of the local population. Welsh LHGs and Scottish LHCCs will be similarly responsible, though LHCCs will not commission health services.

Commissioning services

Each PCO is responsible for the commissioning of health care for a population of 50,000 to 250,000, representing between 10 and 20 general practices. Although commissioning of care remains primary-care led, and therefore benefits from the view of those closest to the patients, it is without the paperchase and bureaucracy of fundholding, and with a much more explicit involvement of the nursing and social perspectives of health care.

Developing services

In addition to commissioning health, each PCO is responsible for monitoring performance and quality (via clinical governance and service agreements), health promotion of the local population, and integration of primary and community care and of primary and secondary care.

A much closer relationship with social services is envisaged such that there is integration between social and health care. Child protection has been especially highlighted as an area where such collaborative working would improve the health of patients and communities (Department of Health 1998a).

Improving the health of the local population

Each PCO will also contribute to the county wide Health Improvement Programme (HImP), which is the local strategy for improving health and health care. The Health Authority has the lead for drawing this up, but is in equal partnership with NHS trusts, PCOs, Local Government and proxy members of the public (represented by voluntary organizations and the Community Health Council (CHC)).

How PCGs and PCTs are organized

Each PCG has a Board, consisting of up to seven GPs (elected by the local general practice community), a lay member (appointed by the Health Authority), two community nurses (who must be clinicians) a Local Authority representative (appointed by social services) and a Heath Authority representative. The Chief Executive of the PCG also has a seat on the board. The chair of the Board may be a doctor, or a nurse or a lay member.

The structure of PCTs is much more complicated. The PCT Management Board has ten members and a chair. The chair must be a lay person. Five of the members are lay and appointed by the Secretary of State (advised by the Health Authority) and five are professional. The professionals on the Management Board are drawn from the Executive Committee of the PCT and are the Chief executive of the PCT, the finance director of the PCT, the chair of the Executive Committee and two health professional members of the Executive Committee. The Management Board is accountable to the Health Authority.

The Executive Committee has up to ten health professionals in addition to the Chief Executive of the PCT, the finance director of the PCT, a social services representative and a chair. The Executive Committee advises the Management Committee and has a responsibility to consult and be accountable to the public. The views of the public, community nursing and social services are therefore specifically sought at board level in the delivery and planning of health care and this is especially so in the case of PCTs. In addition to employed executives, many PCOs have an attached information, Health Promotion and

Public Health specialist, employed by the Health Authority but commissioned by the PCO, giving a broad view on issues of the health needs of the population the PCO serves.

As well as regular full board meetings, subgroups representing, for example, child and family services meet and feed back to the board. In this way, important social issues impacting on health, such as child abuse and domestic violence, are included in the PCO's health care planning.

Change within primary care

The NHS is and will remain primary-care led. A major area of reform in the NHS is in accountability for quality. The mechanisms for ensuring accountability are clinical governance and accountability agreements. Additionally, services must now aim to integrate not just primary and secondary care, but also integrate local authority and primary care. The vehicle for integration is the HImP.

Clinical governance

Clinical governance is a term used to capture a range of activities which occur or will occur, UK wide and throughout the NHS, to ensure and monitor quality. Clinical governance obliges everyone working in the NHS to think about, strive for and monitor quality, to be accountable for quality and to be collectively accountable for the quality of others. The focus for supporting clinical governance within primary care is the PCO (Rosen 2000) (LHG in Wales and LHCC in Scotland). Clinical governance is defined as 'a framework through which NHS organizations are accountable for continuously improving the quality of their services and safeguarding high standards of care by creating an environment in which excellence in clinical care will flourish' (Department of Health 1998b). The approach is expected to apply to improving services, anticipating problems and setting standards. With a commitment to governance comes a commitment to life-long learning and a commitment to tackling poor performance when discovered. Clinical governance is a collective activity. The principles of clinical governance apply to all those who provide or manage patient care services in the NHS. They apply to clinicians and managers alike at both individual and health care organization level, and rest on the axiom that individual failure of performance reflects a wider system failure (Huntington *et al.* 2000).

Accountability

At the 'heart of the concept of clinical governance' is accountability (Allen 2000). Professionals will and always have been accountable to the patients they treat and to their professional organizations, such as the GMC in the case of doctors and the UKCC in the case of nurses. Clinical governance will make these professionals additionally responsible to the local Health Authority, the local community the PCO serves and to peers in the PCO to which they belong (Figure 18.1). A PCO is accountable upwards to the Health Authority, downwards to the population it serves and horizontally to the members of the PCO.

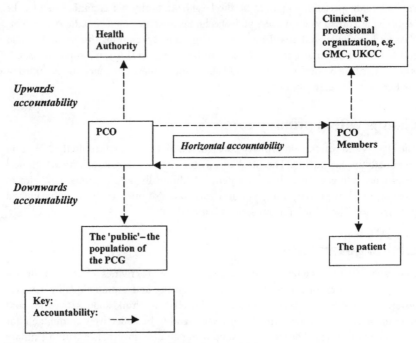

Figure 18.1 Professional accountability in the new NHS.
Reproduced with the permission of the BMJ Publishing Group from Allen (2000).

PCOs are accountable to the Health Authority (upwards accountability)

PCOs have statutory accountability to Health Authorities through Accountability Agreements. In their turn, Heath Authorities are statutorily accountable to Regional Offices of the NHS Executive. Local Authorities, Health Authorities, NHS Trusts, the public and PCOs contribute to and are linked by the HImP.

Accountability agreements

These are between the Health Authority and the PCO. The content is agreed between the Health Authority and the PCO yearly and is used to monitor the performance of the PCO throughout the year. The content of the Accountability Agreement refers to and is partly based on the content of the HImP. The approach of Health Authorities is at the moment an enabling one which assists the PCG to progress, gradually taking up more responsibility en route to becoming a PCT (Department of Health 1999a). However, ultimately, the autonomy of PCOs is earned. Accountability Agreements have teeth; the Health Authority can take back areas of control from PCOs performing poorly.

The HImP

Since the 1990 NHS Act, Health Authorities have been obliged to assess the needs of their population and to use this information to set priorities to improve health. Now, in equal partnership with Local Authorities, NHS Trusts, the public (represented by representative patients groups, voluntary organizations and the CHC) and the PCOs, the Health Authority has responsibility for drawing up a HImP (Figure 18.2). This programme, designed to run over three years but revised yearly, sets out the framework within which all local NHS bodies and all Local Government bodies will operate in order to improve the health and the health services for the population of that county.

The HImP responds to national and local health needs. Nationally, those set out in the White Paper, *Saving Lives, Our Healthier Nation* are to do with the reduction in mortality from heart disease and stroke, accidents, cancer and mental health (Department of Health 1999b). The HImP will also identify local priorities. For example, in 1999, Cambridgeshire identified the need to improve child protection

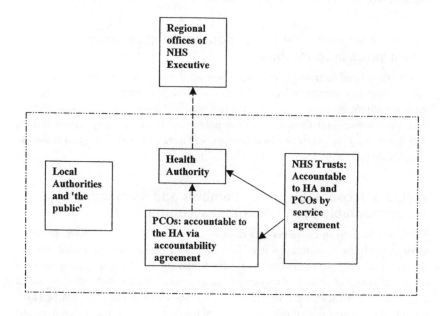

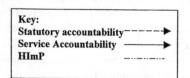

Figure 18.2 Accountability and the HImP.
Reproduced with the permission of The Stationery Office from Department of Health (1997).

services as part of a county-wide initiative to improve the health of children in need. The mechanisms for this were organizational (for example, links between adult mental health and child protection services were improved) and educational (for example, some of the issues around GP education in child protection were addressed).

In addition to national and county-wide priorities, each PCO may also choose one or two very local priorities it has identified. For example, within the Cambridgeshire HImP, mental health was identified as a priority area. One Cambridgeshire PCO with a very dispersed and rural population chose to target this priority around family support, especially that to mothers and their children and in particular, highlighted the problem of family violence.

Each PCO is required to respond to the HImP and set it within the local context of its population, the local financial and managerial capacity and the viewpoint of local partners. The Accountability Agreement between the PCO and the Health Authority refers to the HImP and requires a response from the PCO to national and local HImP priorities. The broad based and consultative nature of the HImP's creation ensures the health needs of the community and the relationship between social need and medical care are both firmly on the agenda of the PCO.

PCOs are accountable to the population they serve: downwards accountability

PCOs are obliged to have lay representation on their boards, designed to foster an appreciation of community issues. Boards may, if they so wish, co-opt lay members onto other groups, such as governance sub groups. Community nurses, with their very close working relationship with the public and local authority representatives with their social perspective on health issues, will have a pivotal role at board level in contributing to public accountability.

A PCO is accountable to its members and its members are accountable to it: horizontal accountability

PCOs will be focal in implementing clinical governance. Organizationally, the PCO chairperson is the 'responsible officer' for governance issues, and answerable through the Accountability Agreement to the Health Authority. PCOs are obliged to appoint a clinical governance lead, a majority have appointed one or more doctors and a community nurse to lead at board level on governance issues. The exact way in which a PCO relates to and communicates with local practices varies, but a common model is that each practice has lead doctors and nurses for prescribing, annual reports, children's issues, clinical governance and other areas as well. PCO board member will usually also visit practices, arrange regular meetings for its members and communicate with them via newsletters as well as on a one-to-one basis. PCOs which have moved to trust status and taken on responsibility for commissioning and providing community services will have additional responsibilities for communication and close working relationships with trust employees, such as school nurses, district nurses and health visitors.

Change within child protection

Diagnosing and managing child abuse has been likened to doing a giant jigsaw puzzle to which participants bring varying numbers and sizes of pieces. The process is therefore cooperative and should, amongst other relationships, involve close, cooperative working relationships within health and between health and social care (Department of Health 1999c). The position of general practitioners, 'long regarded as unsatisfactory by the other professionals' (Stevenson 1998) has been one of relative unengagement and lack of interest in cooperative working (Birchall and Hallett 1995), though there is some encouraging evidence that this may be changing (Bannon *et al.* 1999a). Failure of the child protection system is related not just to failure of diagnosis, but also failure of communication, procedure and record keeping (Reder *et al.* 1993). In other words, failure represents a system failure. Quality in child protection is a whole primary care team and therefore a whole PCO concern. It involves both professional and administrative staff, and is organization-wide; it is a clinical governance issue.

Each of the Health Authority, the 'public', and the PCO has a role in ensuring quality as it relates to child protection (Figure 18.3). PCO boards are accountable to the Health Authority, to the population they serve and to their members. Additionally, the PCO members are accountable to the PCO.

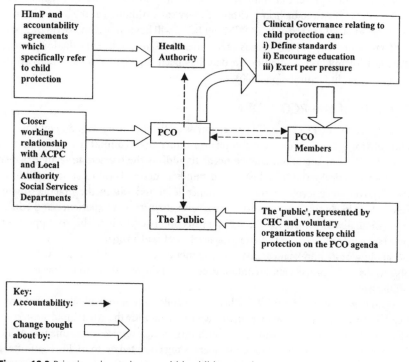

Figure 18.3 Bringing about change within child protection.

The role of the Health Authority as it relates to child protection: upwards accountability

Child protection issues will have to compete for attention at board level. PCO boards will not be short of activity and unless there is outside pressure to do so, it is unlikely that child protection issues will be prioritized by the PCO board itself. Pressure to put child protection issues on the agenda of PCOs will come from above, that is the Health Authority. Child abuse, with its potentially life-long health implications and cost to the health service is an important public health issue (Smith *et al.* 1995). The HImP, with its public health focus, and the perspectives of both the PCO and social services, is an ideal mechanism for generating change. The priorities of the Health Authority and social services relating to child protection can be put on the PCO agenda through the HImP. Issues such as child protection in the general practice setting, highlighted in the HImP and explicit in the accountability agreements between the Health Authority and the PCO. cannot be ignored by PCOs.

The role of the public: downwards accountability

Lay members of the PCO board are in a particularly good position to hear and respond to the voice of voluntary organizations. As yet, voluntary organizations are not represented directly on PCG boards (Audit Commission 2000). PCT Management Boards are differently structured from PCG boards. They have a majority of lay members, and represent an important opportunity for the voice of organizations, such as the NSPCC, to be heard within primary care. Although at the time of writing (October 2000) there are only 17 PCTs, all PCGs will have to become PCTs by 2004.

So far, a minority of PCO boards have undertaken any public consultation exercise. This lack of public consultation to date has been highlighted as an area needing attention (Audit Commission 2000).

The role of the PCO

Acceptance by the PCO of child protection as a HImP priority with an emphasis on control from above alone risks compliance rather than commitment (Huntington *et al.* 2000). Bringing about change needs to address the barriers to change, which are both practical issues and hearts and minds issues and will exist at board level, board governance level, practice governance level and within the practices themselves. It is likely that community nurses, with their greater experience and education (Birchall and Hallett 1995) in child protection issues will be able to support this process at board level and at practice level, and will probably be less in need of persuading of its importance. Board representatives from social services will also be able to assist the process and maintain pressure on the board not to let this issue slip off the agenda.

As an organization (the PCO), rather than a collection of individuals, general practice has an opportunity for meaningful engagement with the Area Child Protection Committee (ACPC) and with local authority social service departments. ACPC involvement can be by PCO board members being co-opted on to ACPC committees, such as those to do with communication or training. Co-opted members are usefully drawn from both clinicians, such as GPs and community nurses, and officers, such as primary care development officers responsible for children's services. ACPC representation on a sub group of the PCO board, such as child and family services subgroups, is also very valuable for improving cooperative working and aiding communication.

What PCOs can do

A PCO may accept its obligations under the HImP to improve its response to child protection issues, but how then does it turn this into a reality at practice level? There are both practical issues the PCO can address and 'hearts and minds issues', to do with the cultural changes needed to encourage engagement of the primary care team and general practice in particular in child protection issues.

Practical issues

PCO boards have a vital contribution to make in defining standards, encouraging education and exerting peer pressure (Grol 1992) with respect to child protection. PCOs can:

1 Define standards by

- Encouraging individual practices to declare standards, for example by writing a practice protocol. Such a protocol should refer to the standards stated in *Working Together* (Department of Health 1999c) around education, note keeping and recording, communication and knowledge of local procedure. As a first step, each PCO could undertake a survey of issues relevant to child protection procedures among practice teams within its catchment area. Questionnaire is an example of such an exercise that might be performed jointly with Social Services, an example of 'joined-up' working.

- Developing clarity about the GP role in child protection: PCOs can help by working with bodies such as the ACPC in defining the role of the GP in child protection issues and work towards a definition of best practice.

2 Encourage education

- PCOs can define a minimum and a 'best practice' educational standard – for GPs, and for their employees as well as GP registrars, for locums and other non-principals.

- PCO can support educational initiatives: managing change is consuming of time and money and although there will be many calls on the clinical governance budget, highlighting the area of child protection signals its importance to the general practice community.

3 Exert peer pressure, for example by developing PCO wide guidelines. It is known that guidelines are more likely to be implemented if they are designed by the group for whom they are intended. Through their boards, PCOs can produce guidance, for example on writing reports for case conferences and then disseminate this along with existing general practice material, such as child health surveillance educational material.

Questionnaire

This questionnaire relates to your service's experience of Social Services' response and follow up of referrals that relate to child protection matters.

Are you clear about the location of the Advice and Assessment Teams?

Do you know the Duty Office telephone numbers?

Do you know the names of the Advice and Assessment Team Managers?

Are you clear about to whom to address a referral?

Do you know the address of the Social Services Neighbourhood offices?

Do you feel you have been given adequate information about any recent changes in the Children's Division?

Do you feel your service is clear about the threshold for making a referral to Social Services?

From your service's experiences of making referrals do you feel that Social Services differentiates and responds to different levels of need appropriately?

In making referrals to Social Services would you consider the response to be courteous and helpful?

Do you believe that Social Services give a timely response to concerns that you refer? (NB Social Services response times are guided by the *Framework for The Assessment of Children in Need and their Families* Department of Health 2000)

From your experience do you feel that the Social Services' response is generally appropriate?

Does your agency routinely receive feedback from Social Services regarding the outcome of enquiries?

Do you feel that Social Services' response is consistent in relation to the level of need referred?

Do you feel that Social Services effectively facilitates joint working in undertaking child protection work?

Do you believe that your service is routinely asked to participate in strategy meetings?

Do you feel that your agency contribution is effectively facilitated at a Case Conference?

Do you feel that case conferences are chaired in a way that maximises service user participation and inclusion?

How effective do you feel the child protection plans are that are made at a case conference?

Do you feel that the social work assessments respond to and value diversity appropriately?

Questionnaire (continued)

Do you feel that the child protection plans from case conferences respond to and value diversity appropriately?

How effective do you think the current systems are within the district in ensuring the protection of children?

How effective do you think is the current social work practice in ensuring the protection of children?

Winning hearts and minds

However much health service reforms and reorganization present an improved machinery and climate for change, changes agreed at PCO board level, even those accepted as governance issues, will not self-implement. All the social, cultural and individual barriers to change will be firmly in place and will need addressing (Bannon et al. 1999a). Many of these barriers and ways of overcoming them have been discussed already in this book. However, from the entirely pragmatic viewpoint of having been involved in such a hearts and minds exercise, there are matters to do with the approach the PCO takes, and the nature of the educational messages it delivers, which are helpful.

An approach which is constructive and positive

1   A positive, rather than blame approach, works best. For example, pointing out to GPs how few case conferences they attend is, on the whole, counter productive.

2   An educational approach, which takes account of the variability of learning needs (Bannon et al. 1999b) amongst doctors, and takes place in a variety of settings, including practice-based ones, works better than any attempt to force change.

3   An approach founded in reality, which acknowledges difficulties of the child protection process and attempts to address some of these.

4   An approach which uses the strength of the PCO as an organization. PCOs are deliberately constructed as multiprofessional organizations, with nursing, lay and social service perspectives as well as those of the general practitioner. The organization is accountable for quality but its members are accountable to it for the quality of their performance (via clinical governance). These are very positive organisational features for those wishing to see change in child protection.

Education in child protection

The ultimate aim of the PCO should be that everyone working in the PCO has received some sort of child protection education (Figure 18.4). This is considered as a whole practice, *introductory training*, a clinician's, *foundation level* training, and finally, the PCO needs to encourage interested GPs to develop a *special interest* in the subject and be its champion.

Introductory	Foundation	Special interest
Who? All general practitioners and their employees	Who? Clinicians who have contact with children	Who? Clinicians and non clinicians with a special interest- opinion leaders and champions
What: Practice based education	What: part of continuing professional development.	
How: Practice based education adopted as a governance issue by PCOs, which support its development and implementation	How: Peer pressure, PCO leads by example. Professions include child protection in their PDP Practices include child protection education in their PPDP	How: PCOs encourage and supports development e.g. through links with ACPC and PCO child and family sub groups
Outcomes: 1) Better understanding of Role Recognition Referral 2) Practice writes their own child protection protocol	Outcomes: 1) lay the foundations for interdisciplinary working 2) enable clinicians to participate in case conferences, core groups and assessment in more meaningful ways	Outcomes: 1) maintain and promote partnership 2) be a champion, for example drawing attention to the health implications of domestic violence 3) opinion leaders encouraging excellence by challenging current practice and educational standards

Figure 18.4 Framework for training.

Introductory level education for the whole practice team

Child protection is a quality issue, it is a clinical governance issue and it is a whole practice issue. Correct management is not just a question of recognition and referral by clinicians. Responsibilities are administrative and procedural as well as clinical, so appropriate education needs to be considered for the whole team (Glennie and Horwath 2000). Appropriate, *introductory level*, education for non-clinicians is as important as it is for clinicians. It is the GP as the employer who is responsible for the education of the general practice team (Department of Health 1999c). Each person within the general practice team needs to have basic knowledge regarding the importance of child protection issues, their own role within the practice, and an understanding of to whom they should report concerns.

Foundation level education for all clinicians

Foundation level education needs to highlight child protection as a general practice issue in which GPs, as members of the primary health care team, have a vital role. It should also enable the clinician to take part in interdisciplinary working. The importance of the education of other clinicians in the general practice should not be overlooked, in particular, practice nurses risk being marginalised. Ideally, education in child protection should be included within a professional's personal development plan (PDP) (Department of Health 1998c) and linked with the practice professional development plan (PPDP), such that it is seen as a whole practice learning activity aimed at improving practice performance, and hence patient care (Pringle 2000).

Special interest: finding champions

Within each PCO or group of PCOs, doctors, nurses and non clinicians have a vital role in maintaining and promoting partnership between key child protection agencies. As organizations, PCOs have an important opportunity to form new and positive relationships between primary care (and this applies especially to general practice) and social service departments. There is a need for a few PCO members to champion important, but all too easily ignored issues related to child abuse, such as domestic violence. Finally, the PCO needs opinion leaders to challenge current practice and to set new standards and expectations within child protection. Annoying though these individuals may be, they too need cherishing.

Conclusion

Reforms to the NHS are an additional burden to those working in it, and like Rita we might question their usefulness, 'I wonder if I'll ever understand any of it. It's like startin' all over again, y'know with a different language'. What Rita got from her education however, was not just a new language, but a different way of thinking and a mechanism for challenging the accepted norms of her own culture. At their very best, the NHS reforms present us with a different way of thinking and at the least with an improved mechanism for managing change. These latest reforms will not be the last, they are not necessarily the best, they are simply what we have got. Understanding how PCOs work and the system in which they themselves are situated enables pressure for change to be applied at many points within that system from both organizations and individuals, within primary care and outside primary care.

Acknowledgement

Sally Hind, Chief Executive of South Cambs PCG commented most helpfully on an earlier draft of this chapter.

References

Allen P (2000) Accountability for clinical governance: developing collective responsibility for quality in primary care. *British Medical Journal* 321: 608–11.

Audit Commission (2000) The PCG agenda: early progress of primary care groups in 'The New NHS'. London: The Stationery Office.

Bannon M, Carter YH and Ross L (1999a) Perceived barriers to full participation in the child protection process: preliminary conclusions from focus group discussions in West Midlands UK. *Journal of Interprofessional Care* 13: 239–48.

Bannon M, Carter YH, Barwell F and Hicks C (1999b) Perceptions held by general practitioners in England regarding their training needs in child abuse and neglect. *Child Abuse Review* 8: 276–83.

Birchall E and Hallett C (1995) *Working Together in Child Protection*. London: HMSO.

Department of Health (1997) *The New NHS: Modern, Dependable*. London: The Stationery Office.

Department of Health (1998a) *The new NHS Modern and Dependable. Health Service circular*, 1998/065. London: The Stationery Office.

Department of Health (1998b). *A First Class Service. Quality in the new NHS*. London: The Stationery Office.

Department of Health (1998c) *A Review of Continuing Professional Development In General Practice: A Report By The Chief Medical Officer*. London: The Stationery Office.

Department of Health (1999a) *Corporate Governance. Health Service circular*, 1999/048. London: The Stationery Office.

Department of Health (1999b) *Saving Lives: Our Healthier Nation*. London: The Stationery Office.

Department of Health (1999c) *Working Together To Safeguard Children*. London: The Stationery Office.

Department of Health (2000) *The NHS Plan, A Plan For Investment, A Plan For Reform*. London: The Stationery Office.

Glennie S and Horwath J (2000) Inter agency training: broadening the focus. *Child Abuse Review* 9: 148–56.

Grol R (1992) Implementing guidelines in general practice care. *Quality in Health Care* 1: 184–91.

Huntington J, Gillam S and Rosen R (2000) Organisational development for clinical governance. *British Medical Journal* 321: 679–82.

NHS Executive (1998) The New Nhs Modern And Dependable; Establishing Primary Care Groups. *Health Service Circular* 1998/065. London: The Stationery Office.

NHS Wales (1998) Putting patients first. *http://www.wales.nhs.uk/publications/w hitepaper98* (accessed 30.9.00).

Pringle M (2000) Clinical governance in primary care. *British Medical Journal* 321: 737–40.

Reder P, Duncan S and Grey M (1993) *Beyond Blame: Child Abuse Tragedies Revisited*. London: Routledge.

Rosen R (2000) Improving quality in the changing world of primary care. *British Medical Journal* 321: 551–54.

Russell W (1996) *Plays: 1: Breezeblock Park, Our Day Out, Stage and Hens, Educating Rita*. London: Methuen Drama.

SHOW (2000) Scottish health on the web. *http://www.scot.nhs.uk /*(accessed 30.9.00).

Smith D, Pearce L, Pringle M and Caplan R (1995) Adults with a history of child sexual abuse: evaluation of a pilot therapy service. *British Medical Journal* 310: 1175–8.

Stevenson O (1998) *Neglected Children: Issues And Dilemmas*. Oxford: Blackwell.

Chapter 19

The child protection process: an international perspective

Rachael Hetherington

Introduction

First there was child welfare; then the 'battered baby' syndrome; then child abuse; and then child protection. This is roughly how the response of services in this country has developed since the major shifts in structures and services that followed the wartime experiences of the evacuation of children and the subsequent creation of the National Health Service and the welfare state. During the 1950s and 1960s, while the post-war child welfare services were being developed in the UK, research in the US was beginning to establish the knowledge which led to the definition of child abuse (followed by child sexual abuse). This knowledge swiftly became available in the UK and in other European countries, and everywhere began to affect policies and practice in state interventions in families. Development was not uniform in the speed at which it took place, and the nature of developments depended on the systems that already existed. In the UK we have tended to look to the US rather than other European countries for new ideas and approaches and for this reason and because of a shared language, child abuse became a focus of concern earlier in this country than elsewhere. However, by the second half of the 1980s, new legislation on child welfare and child protection was being debated not only in this country, but in most other European countries.

This chapter looks at the ways in which child welfare and child protection services have developed in some other European countries, in order to see what we can learn about the functioning of our system through comparisons.

Why study other systems? The value of making comparisons

The health and welfare services of European countries have broadly similar aims, but their structures and their methods of services delivery vary greatly. Their economic circumstances vary and their choices about state expenditure on welfare lead to different levels of financing. So what can be learnt by studying the health and welfare systems of other countries that is useful for practitioners in these services in this country? We practice within the laws and procedures of our own country, and we may question the relevance of learning how other people organize these matters. However, this learning is potentially useful in several ways. At a time of increasing mobility between countries, practitioners may need to know about the services and systems of other countries in order to ensure the protection of children whose families may be moving abroad. There may also be new ideas about services and good practice which are transferable from one country to another. Most importantly, we can learn more about how we work ourselves, and about the structures within which we work, and how they affect what we can do. We can develop new perspectives on our own practice and begin to understand it differently.

Our initial motivation for looking to other European countries was a feeling of frustration and anxiety about the way in which the UK, and more specifically the English, child protection system was developing. As a result of the research process described below, we began to see the English system as problematic in certain specific ways, and to identify some of the underlying reasons.

The research on which the chapter is based

Rationale and method

The research started with a comparison between child protection practice in England and in France (Hetherington 1994; Cooper et al. 1995). It was later extended to include four other European countries (Hetherington et al. 1997). We studied altogether six systems because Belgium has different systems for the French and the Flemish speaking communities, and Scotland has a different system from England and Wales. The scope of the project was widened to include a small study of parents' experience of child welfare procedures in three countries (Baistow and Hetherington 1998; Baistow and Wilford 2000). Recently a cross-country comparison looking at inter-agency cooperation for children with a mentally ill parent has been completed (Hetherington et al. 2000; Hetherington et al. 2001). This last project, which looked at community mental health services as well as child welfare, produced information on the wider topics of child neglect, preventive work and mental health promotion.

The method of study was based on working with the people who, as professionals or parents, were stakeholders in the system. The aim was to find out not only how the systems were supposed to work, but how they actually worked in practice. The research projects into child protection and into children with mentally ill parents took as their point of departure a case vignette which was studied by professionals in all the countries, who then suggested what would happen in that situation in their country. They discussed what action would be taken, what resources were available, what laws and services were involved. They were also asked why they would make the decisions that they did and what theories they were using.

The research with parents took a rather different form. Parents who had had some experience of their country's child welfare system (not necessarily child protection) were asked about that experience. The interviews were unstructured, and the numbers were small, so their views were not statistically analysable, but their experiences demonstrated how the different welfare systems responded to some of the people for whose help they were designed.

Findings

By comparing the different responses to the same case situation in the first research project, we identified differences in structures and child protection practice between the different countries.

The legal system

Within the UK, the legal child protection system in Scotland is significantly different from the system of England and Wales, and Northern Ireland. In the first research project all our practitioner groups were English, so these comments relate specifically to England. We found that England had a very different legal system for child protection from the other countries studied.

In all the other countries studied, cases of child protection and cases of juvenile crime are heard in the same court. This demonstrates an approach to children's problems that regards children's behaviour as responsive to social and family situations rather than seeing children as either victims or victimizers. The principle on which the judicial system is organized in other countries is 'inquisitorial' rather than 'adversarial'. This means that the judge for children is in charge of the investigation of a situation, rather than social workers. The judge for children is able to require police to investigate, if there may be a criminal charge to be made against the parents, and can ask social workers to make an assessment, or ask for specialist reports. These matters are not the responsibility of the professionals in health or social services (except in providing an assessment when required to do so), and they are not therefore put in the position of making accusations against parents. The grounds for compulsory intervention in families are more widely drawn. For example, in France the judge for children can make an order for 'help in upbringing', 'if the safety or morality of a minor are in danger, or if the conditions of his upbringing are seriously compromised' (Civil Code article 375). In the Flemish community of Belgium, the grounds are that a child is in 'a problematic upbringing situation: a condition, in which the physical integrity, the affective, moral intellectual or social developmental chances of the minors are negatively affected due to special event, relational conflicts or the circumstances in which they live,' and that work on a voluntary basis has failed or is not possible (Pieck undated). These broad grounds are based on an underlying expectation that the state is concerned not only with child protection but with child welfare.

None of the countries (except for Scotland, which has the same area child protection committee system as the rest of the UK) has a child protection register or a child protection conference system. They took cases before the court more readily than in England, and used more supervision orders.

Compared with other countries, the English system was inflexible. Social workers from other countries were very impressed by the way in which child protection conferences were run and by the standard of the social work reports that were presented at them. But they were concerned about the levels of bureaucracy of the English system and the lack of autonomy of the workers. At the same time, they were quite shocked by the amount of power given to the English social work department by a child care order, and by the fact that the order had no time limit, and was not automatically reviewed by the courts.

Professional time

English social workers commented on the number of social workers available in other countries and the amount of time that they could give to the families that they worked with. Germany was seen as particularly fortunate, in that they had specialist family support teams, staffed by qualified family social workers who could work intensively with a family if necessary visiting several times a week, and undertaking practical tasks along side the family in order to develop a working relationship and teach through doing together. In France there were similar workers, and though the levels of support available were not as high as in Germany (and the Netherlands), there was still more than in England. As a result, more preventive work could be undertaken and supervision orders could be effectively implemented.

Risk

English social workers placed more emphasis on risk and dangerousness. Having fewer resources for family support, English social workers had little option than to be focused on assessing risk and danger. Social workers in other European countries who could be more easily involved at an earlier stage in the development of family problems, and who could more easily have the backing of the court, had less need to concentrate on the evaluation of risk. Because of the greater availability of professional time, in a crisis, they were more likely already to know the family. They were often impressed by the clarity of the English social workers in identifying and categorizing risk, but felt that this could get in the way of more positive approaches. French and German social workers were prepared to continue to work with families where English social workers felt that they would have had to call a child protection conference and initiate child protection procedures, which would, at least for a time, have made constructive work with the family extremely difficult (Cooper and Hetherington 1999).

The balance of advantages

Social workers in other countries saw some benefits to the English system, but many problems. A group of social workers in Italy took part in the first research project which was on child protection. One of the Italian social workers felt that the English child protection system, the register, the conference and the judicial system would have been helpful in dealing with an extremely conservative judiciary and a powerful patriarchal family system. A group of social workers in what had been East Germany thought that the English system reminded them of their old system under the communist regime. Even allowing for possible distortions in their understanding of another system, these reactions were a striking commentary on the rigidity of the

English system, and the fact that such a framework could be seen, depending on circumstances, as an asset or a problem.

Social workers in England saw many advantages in other systems. Although there were aspects of the English system that were important to them, they found much that they preferred in other countries. Although there were important differences in the systems of the other countries, English social workers identified similarities between other European systems which they thought were advantageous. They saw the other systems as offering greater flexibility and avoiding the need to take on a role of investigator. The judicial system in France and in other countries took the responsibility for outlining the failures of the parents from the social workers. In some respects the powers of the judge for children made social workers less powerful, but at the same time it paradoxically seemed to give them more authority, because the social workers felt that they were supported by the power of the judge. This was attractive to the English social workers who saw French social workers as less isolated and less at risk of blame than themselves. The response was striking, because the French social worker in the local authority social services department can be prosecuted for failing to refer a case to the judge, so that system is not without its threats for French practitioners.

What lies behind the findings

These differences in systems and in the workers' experience of their systems have complex origins.

Differences in expectations

There seemed to be different expectations of the family. In all the countries that we have studied (in northern and southern Europe) the family seems to be a more solid structure than in England; there was even some difference in this within the UK between England, Northern Ireland and Scotland. The difference is demonstrated by the sustained efforts made by social workers, and supported by the legal system, to return children to their families. French and German social workers were more ready to take children into care, but expected them to return home, and continued to work at this over years. It was not expected that taking children into care would lead to the disintegration of the family. This was also evident in differences in the law and in attitudes to adoption. Adoption against the wishes of the parents is scarcely possible, and the adoption of older children is very unusual. Altogether the family is seen as less fragile.

There are also different expectations of the relationship between the family and the state (and therefore between social workers and the family). Many European countries have something equivalent to the French Civil Code which sets out the ground rules for citizenship. There is a social contract between the state and the citizen which implies that the state has a right and a duty to intervene and to offer help in the proper upbringing of children, who are the future citizens. The parents have a reciprocal right to help. The majority of EU countries now have mandatory reporting of child abuse (although this can mean very different things in different countries, depending on who has to report, and what level of concern has to be reported). An increasing number have 'no smacking' laws.

These differences are important because they affect expectations of the relationship between the law, professionals and the family. In child protection, social workers and other professionals who take up any official position in relation to the family do so as representatives of the state (however much they wish to distance themselves from this). In France, and in general in continental European countries (the position in the Nordic countries is slightly different) the judge for children represents the child. The social workers derive their authority from the judge for children, and are thus acting for the child. As noted above, the grounds for intervention are widely drawn.

Differences in structures

There is no consistent pattern of service structures across Europe. The most important variables are the organization of the health services, the division and sharing of service delivery between voluntary agencies and local authority services and the nature of the legal system. Although all European countries have a compulsory health service, some of the services are organized on an insurance principle, where citizens pay at point of use and reclaim their payment (or a proportion of their payment) later. Some are, as in the UK, free at point of use. Community maternal and child health systems vary considerably in where they are located and how full a universal system is provided. The Nordic countries have very few voluntary agencies involved in the delivery of child protection and child welfare services (in Sweden and Denmark, virtually none). Germany, the Netherlands and Belgium have many. This affects the experience of the families, who have more choice in the latter group of countries, but a better 'safety net' in the Nordic countries.

As has already been described, England and Wales and Northern Ireland are alone in having an adversarial legal system, and in separating child protection from juvenile crime. This is possibly the major determinant of the experience of families where children are being protected. An adversarial system sets up a culture of blame, and the need to provide evidence of significant harm dominates English social work procedure from the earliest point of intervention. The nature of the legal system has a profound effect on the processes of child protection.

Differences in resources

It appeared that resources in other countries were greater. This may have been partly because they were differently distributed. The resources of the child protection and child welfare system in England and Wales are focused on the 'heavy end' of the work. It is much harder here to find resources for preventive work and early intervention, while it is accepted that resources should be made available for expert reports for court hearings, extensive social work reports and the guardian *ad litem* system. Even allowing for this, our researches seemed to show that in a number of ways other countries put more resources into child welfare. There is more provision for the family support services of family workers and family aides, and the work is more likely to be undertaken by qualified workers. In many countries there is almost universal nursery school provision for children over three, and easily available provision for children over two and a half (Bradshaw *et al.* 1993). Financial benefits in support of families (such as family allowances) are more generous, and the universal maternal and child health services are better funded, (although not all countries have this service). It is also well documented that health services in this country are under-resourced compared with most other European countries.

One of the most noticeable differences in resourcing that emerged from the comparative studies was the difference in the amount of time that professionals of all disciplines had for their work. Social workers, health visitors, and GPs in this country all seem to work under a pressure of time much greater than elsewhere. This was made very clear in the study comparing parental experience of child welfare systems. In the three countries studied, France, Germany and England, the parents were united in valuing very highly time spent in listening to their problems and in supporting them in their negotiations with other services. It was more difficult for the English parents to get this time than for the French or German.

The place of primary care professionals in other countries

Not all countries have the same concept of the primary health care team. In countries with an insurance-based health service such as Germany, there is no real equivalent to the GP. The family may choose to have a 'family doctor' who they use in the same way as a GP, but they can choose to go directly to a specialist. On the other hand, in northern Italy where some of our research took place, the equivalent to the GP, the '*medico di base*' has a very important position, and is a link between specialist services and the community. But in the Nordic countries which all had a state delivered medical service, we found that the GP did not necessarily have the central role that is expected here. The maternal and child health services vary considerably in where they are located. In Germany, with an insurance-based medical system and a low level of direct state provision of services, maternal and child health services tend to be provided by non-governmental agencies and to be available on the insurance (and therefore not a universal service). In France, the maternal and child health service is well resourced and is an important part of the local authority social service. The joint multidisciplinary area team of maternal and child health workers and social workers is a very important aspect of the French child protection system. It enables the easy sharing of information between workers who are used to working together and have developed ways of doing this. In Sweden and Denmark, there is a similar pattern. In northern Italy yet other structures have been developed, and the '*Consultorio Familiare*' provides a maternal and child health service based in the health service rather than local government, but employing social workers and psychologists as well as doctors and health visitors. The location of health visitors and social workers in relation to each other has an important effect on the liaison and cooperation between the two services, and more widely on the connections that are made between universal and targeted services. The countries in our study that did not have a state-run universal maternal and child health service envied those that did.

Our most recent research, which has looked at cooperation between agencies and services for families with a mentally ill parent, showed the great importance of the primary care services as a safety net and a potential source of information about families where there are significant difficulties which have not yet reached the level of child protection issues, but which urgently need preventive work and social support. The UK system seemed to have great potential in this respect, but to be handicapped by lack of resources; perhaps the most important of these resources was time.

The English system through other eyes

To summarize, other countries, whatever the differences between their systems – and there has not been space in this chapter to do more than indicate these differences – saw the English system as bureaucratic, with an over-emphasis on administrative and legal procedures. In their eyes, although the law was not necessarily used more in England, the legal process dominated intervention. Action was restricted to rescue and monitoring, and the system discouraged early intervention with the aim of prevention.

In a useful collection of accounts of child protections systems from Europe and North America, Neil Gilbert (1997) initially categorized the systems as those that had mandatory reporting of child abuse and those that did not. He found that the significant categorization was not between having or not having mandatory reporting, but between a focus on family support or child protection. He categorized the Nordic countries and the northern European countries (Germany, the Netherlands and Belgium) as focusing on family support, and the English speaking countries (the US, Canada and England) as focusing on child protection. Our research supported this categorization. France and Italy, although considerably different in approach from the Nordic and northern European countries, shared the same proactive approach to support both at the universal level of benefits and nursery school provision, and in their expectation that the role of the social services (and therefore the state) was to support families and not only to monitor them.

Conclusions: what do comparisons suggest about the English system

In comparison with other countries in Europe, the aims of the English system are very restricted. The basis of intervention is defined as 'being in need', not 'wanting help'. The parents who told us about their experience in France and Germany approached services asking for help with an expectation that they would be heard. The parents in England had very low expectations of getting help, and felt that they had to demonstrate not only that in their own eyes they needed help, but that their child might be 'at risk'. Being on the child protection register was the only sure way of getting help.

This may be partly a matter of resources, but that is not a complete explanation. It is not just a refusal to spend money; we spend a great deal on the court process. It seems to be a more fundamental problem connected to a wish not to interfere, to respect the right to be left alone. It demonstrates an attitude that says that the state should keep out of family life. The family is best left to sort itself out unless 'significant harm' to the child can be proved. This is likely to mean that intervention has to be delayed until the situation has deteriorated. It makes preventive work difficult, often impossible.

This right to non-intervention is perpetually in conflict with the right of the child to be heard and to be protected. All professionals working with children are caught up in this conflict, and the primary care professionals are often the people who know most clearly that intervention will be needed, and are unable to do anything until things have got worse. 'Monitoring' a family without time or resources to take any steps to alter the behaviours that are being monitored is frustrating and wasteful of resources and opportunities. Assessments of 'need' that are not backed by the resources to meet those needs create anger and disillusionment. It is particularly hard for workers in the universal services (such as primary care professionals and teachers) who can see that a little help at an early stage might prevent problems from developing, but who know from experience that social services are not able to offer this help.

In this climate, English professionals are pessimistic, and social workers often assume that their intervention is not wanted. The parents we talked to thought otherwise; they wanted help, and their anger was at the lack of support and work to prevent crises. Working with families in difficulties is never easy, and quite properly raises anxieties in professionals in all countries, but elsewhere in Europe there was not the same level of dissatisfaction with the system. The philosophy of non-intervention seems to have led to a focus on rescue rather than prevention which is then supported by an adversarial legal process; these elements combine to create a system that may be efficient in protecting from further harm but which is ineffective in preventing harm. It is not without good reason that, in England, many people working in the field of child protection feel not only anxious, but helpless and frustrated.

References

Baistow K and Hetherington R (1998) Parents' experiences of child welfare interventions: an Anglo-French comparison. *Children and Society* 12: 113–24.

Baistow K and Wilford G (2000) Parents' experiences of child welfare interventions: an Anglo-German comparison. *Children and Society* 14: 343–54.

Bradshaw J and Ditch J (1993) *Support For Children: A Comparison Of Arrangements In Fifteen Countries*. London: HMSO.

Cooper A, Hetherington R, Baistow K, Pitts J and Spriggs S (1995) *Positive Child Protection: A View from Abroad*. Lyme Regis: Russell House Publishing.

Cooper A and Hetherington R (1999) Negotiation, in N Parton, C Wattam (eds) *Child Sexual Abuse: Responding to the Experiences of Children*. Chichester: John Wiley and Sons.

Gilbert N (ed.) (1997) *Combatting Child Abuse: International Perspectives and Trends*. Oxford: Oxford University Press.

Hetherington R (1994) Trans-manche partnerships. *Adoption and Fostering* 18(3): 17–21.

Hetherington R, Cooper A, Smith P and Wilford G (1997) *Protecting Children: Messages from Europe*. Lyme Regis: Russell House Publishing.

Hetherington R, Baistow K, Johanson P and Mesie J (2000) *Professional Interventions for Mentally Ill Parents and their Children: Building a European Model. Final Report on the Icarus Project*. London: Centre for Comparative Social Work Studies, Brunel University.

Hetherington R, Baistow K, Katz I, Mesie J and Trowell J (2001) *The Welfare of Children with a Mentally Ill Parent: Learning from Inter-country Comparisons*. Chichester: John Wiley and Sons.

Pieck A (undated) *Special Youth Assistance in Flanders*. Brussels: Ministry of the Flemish Community.

Chapter 20

Prevention: current and future trends

Kevin D. Browne and Catherine E. Hamilton

Introduction

The contents of this book reflect the debate about what services can be delivered in order to prevent child abuse and neglect and ameliorate the traumatic consequences for victims of child maltreatment. Most authors conclude that a multisector, inter-disciplinary approach is the most effective way of working together to provide protection to children (Hallett and Birchell 1992; Department of Health 1995, 1999). Indeed, guidelines have been published by the Department of Health (1999) on how a range of professionals can work together to safeguard children.

The aims of this chapter are to consider the future of child protection, and suggest ways in which prevention of child abuse and neglect can be enhanced by adopting a more holistic public health approach.

The public health approach

The World Health Organisation (1998a, 1999a) defines a public health approach as the viewing of child abuse and neglect within the broader context of child welfare, families and communities. From a health service perspective, this requires the integration of best practices within three areas of service provision to families and children: safe pregnancy and childbirth, the management of childhood health and illness, and targeting services for families who have a high number of risk factors associated with child abuse and neglect.

Safe pregnancy and childbirth

The following guidelines are adapted from the World Health Organisation (1998b):

- Pre-birth: prenatal screening of the foetus for abnormalities (using ultrasound) and the promotion of healthy lifestyles in the mother in order to protect the foetus (e.g. reducing maternal substance misuse, managing physical and mental illness).

- During birth: the promotion of natural delivery and the use of appropriate technology. Encouraging significant others (usually the father) to be present to support the mother and skin contact between mother and baby immediately following birth. This promotes positive birth experiences for parents which, in turn, encourages parental bonding to the infant.

◆ After birth: 24-hour access of significant others to the mother and child in the maternity unit, appropriate neonatal care and advice on practical parenting skills (e.g. breastfeeding, bathing, etc.). Promotion of sensitive parenting through positive post-birth experiences.

Midwifery nurses are best placed to provide continuity of care to pregnant mothers. This involves the same midwife offering individualized support with pre-birth home visits, assistance in childbirth and infant care throughout pregnancy until 10 days after birth. This is regarded as the 'best practice' model for promoting natural child-birth and parental bonding. In terms of child protection, such an approach increases the likelihood of positive parenting and thereby limits the possibility of infant abandonment, poor parenting and attachment, abuse and neglect.

Integrated management of childhood health and illness

The management of child health and illness by primary health care teams and community health professionals is aimed at the prevention of child disability, morbidity and mortality, as well as at limiting the stress to parents in caring for a sick child. However, children coming to the attention of health services through home or clinic visits also offer the potential to screen for the possibility of maltreatment.

All children coming into contact with the health service can be observed and checked in the normal way for physical injuries and illnesses. During the examination, the possibility of non-accidental injury and illnesses occurring because of abuse and/or neglect should be kept in mind. In the absence of a standardized screening tool, history taking by doctors and nurses on the condition of the child should include the following components to promote identification of and protection from child abuse and neglect:

◆ History of family circumstances (e.g. presence of isolation, violence, addiction or mental illness)

◆ History of child's condition (e.g. story doesn't explain injury, delay in seeking help)

◆ Child's physical condition when undressed (e.g. presence of disability, lesions or genital discharge)

◆ Child's physical care (e.g. cleanliness, teeth, hair, nails, hygiene)

◆ Child's behaviour (e.g. frozen hyper-vigilance or aggressive hyperactivity)

◆ Parents/caretaker's behaviour and demeanour (e.g. low self-esteem, depressed, over anxious, insensitive, careless, punishing, defensive).

A standardized screening tool which is in common use in emergency rooms of hospitals in Holland is reproduced in Appendix 1, as an example of how child protection can be incorporated into health service provision for families and children.

Child protection

It is suggested that Child Protection Services should focus on preventative and protective strategies, offering interventions to families with a high number risk factors associated with child abuse and neglect. If possible, the services should be targeted to these families before maltreatment begins. According to the Department of Health, Department of Education and Employment and the Home Office (2000), Health and Social Services should assess families in the following holistic way:

- Assessment of children's development needs in general;
- Assessment of the parent(s) capacity to respond appropriately to their child's needs;
- Assessment of the wider social and environmental factors that impact on the capacity to parent.

This is known as the 'Lilac Book' assessment format. Risk factors are identified from 'undesirable' characteristics associated with the child, the parents and the family environment. When the number and severity of risk factors present pass a threshold, child protection services are automatically offered. However, it is important not to stigmatise families who have yet to harm their child(ren) and targeting these families should be based on the principle of priority for services. Therefore, families should be considered as 'high priority' or 'low priority' for services rather than regarded as 'high risk' or 'low risk' for child abuse and neglect.

Advantages of early intervention

The importance of early intervention can be considered from two, very different perspectives: the impact on the child victims and the financial cost to society.

Looking at victimization, younger children are particularly vulnerable to abuse and/or neglect. Indeed, in 2000 the highest rate of registration on the Child Protection Register in England and Wales was for physical abuse and neglect in young children under one year – 71 per 10,000 (Department of Health 2000). Furthermore, rates of infant death across different populations highlight the risk to young children. Child abuse and neglect is one of the most common causes of death and disability to children under 5 years, although the risk of being a victim of murder or disability is greatest in a first year of life. Parents are the most common offenders. Despite a bias to find natural causes for infant death, it is estimated that in the United Kingdom two children per week die from maltreatment (5 in 100,000 births). This compares to four children per week in Australia (10 in 100,000 births) and 16 children per week in the USA (40 in 100,000 births). Similar rates have been found for each country in terms of children disabled for life through abuse and neglect as an infant (Browne and Lynch 1995). Therefore, it is essential that prediction and prevention occur from birth.

The financial costs of child abuse and neglect include both costs for the short and long-term treatment of victims and the less apparent impact on other areas of society. The World Health Organisation (1999a) highlighted a number of areas for inclusion in calculations of cost. These were medical care for victims, mental health provision for victims, legal costs for public child care, criminal justice and prosecution costs, treatment of offenders, social work provision and specialist education. Overall, it has been estimated that the total economic cost in the United Kingdom is £735 million pounds per annum, compared to $12,410 million dollars per annum in the USA (National Commission of Enquiry for the Prevention of Child Abuse 1996; WHO 1999a).

The incredible cost of child protection once child abuse and neglect has occurred justifies more expenditure on preventative measures and services to support children and their families.

Prevention of child abuse and neglect

Strategies for the prevention of child maltreatment fall into three categories: primary (at the whole population), secondary (targeting groups) and tertiary (after maltreatment has occurred).

Primary prevention

Primary prevention is aimed at the whole population. Teachers, GPs, practice nurses, health visitors and nursery workers are all important in providing appropriate advice and support. For example, community nurses (health visitors) have ongoing contact with all children under 5 in terms of providing advice on practical parenting skills, health and parental well-being.

Primary prevention services offered to everyone within the population include home visits by health workers, education of parents and caregivers, school programmes on parenting and child development, day nursery places, telephone helplines and drop-in community centres. The purpose of this support is to assist positive parenting skills and to encourage the development of a secure attachment between parent and child. Secure attachments are highly significant in the early prevention of child maltreatment, first, because of the long-term positive impact on child development it engenders (e.g. positive self-image). Second, in situations where a high number of risk factors for child maltreatment are present, child abuse and neglect are more likely to occur in the absence of secure, positive attachments (Morton and Browne 1998).

Many initiatives aimed at promoting positive parenting now exist (Sure Start in England; Triple P in Australia). However, other strategies can be used regularly by primary health professionals, even in the absence of a full programme. Promoting positive parenting skills and sensitivity can be achieved in a fairly straightforward manner by raising awareness of verbal abuse and the implications of this on the development of a positive self-image in the child (see Table 20.1).

From a public health perspective, prevention begins with professional awareness of such issues as the mental health needs of the parent(s), negative aspects of perinatal care and the importance of secure attachments. In turn, primary care professionals can utilize this information in their work with parents and pass on appropriate knowledge to those parents. For example, information on how to cope with post-natal depression, the dangers of shaking or roughly handling a newborn or educating parents about the development of attachment processes.

Table 20.1 Primary prevention by promoting positive parenting

Harsh words hurt	Kind words help
Shut up	Please
Stop it	Well done
Go away	You're clever
You're stupid	You're good
You're bad	I love you
Wish you were never born	

The development of secure attachments, being complex, will be considered in more detail. The importance of imparting knowledge of this process to parents is to assist them in understanding the needs of their child and temperamental differences. For the purposes of parental understanding, this can be separated into three stages.

♦ Birth: parent to infant bonding is a result of the psychological availability of the parent and the genetic predispositions of the child to respond to the parent. This may occur immediately after birth or take some time to develop within the first six months (see Sluckin et al. 1983).

♦ 5–12 months: formulation of infant to parent bond (infant attachment) with maturity where the child shows a preference for the primary caregiver, demonstrates some distress when left by the primary caregiver and is comforted by the presence of the primary caregiver. The infant uses the primary caregiver as a base for exploration and as a source of imitation (see Bowlby 1969).

♦ 12–24 months: infant attachment quality (secure/insecure) is measurable and observable, and can be classified into (a) insecure and avoidant, (b1) secure and independent, (b2) secure and dependent, (c) insecure and ambivalent, (d) disorganized (see Browne and Saqi 1988b; Morton and Browne 1998).

It is important, however, for professionals to remain aware that, whilst providing simple explanations to parents might assist in development of attachment, the assessment of attachment is not simplistic and requires appropriate training. A common misperception is to refer to a child as 'attached'. Nearly all children are attached in some form, it is the quality of infant attachment which is of interest, i.e., secure or insecure. Maccoby (1980) describes how the quality of attachment in a child is dependent on the levels of acceptance, accessibility, consistency, sensitivity and cooperation of the primary caregiver (usually the natural mother). Whilst at times this can appear to be 'common sense', it does not *always* follow that a maltreated child is insecurely attached, nor that a child who clings to their mother is securely attached. However, it is more common for maltreated, abused and neglected children to be less securely attached and usually show patterns of insecurity and anti-social stranger anxiety. Indeed, a meta-analysis of 13 studies showed insecure attachment to the mother in 76% of maltreated samples compared to 34% of non-maltreated samples (Morton and Browne 1998). The long-term consequences of an insecure attachment in early childhood have now been clearly recognised and described. They may be summarized as follows (Cassidy and Shaver 1999; Simpson and Rholes 1998; Solomon and George 1999):

- The early carer–infant relationship is internalized by the child and may be the 'prototype' or 'model' to which all future relationships are assimilated and are based upon;
- The child is likely to develop an image of him/herself as unworthy of love and affection and lacking control over his/her environment;
- Maltreated, abused and neglected children may have greater problems forming relationships with siblings, peers, intimate partners and their own children in future.

It is important to recognize that the transition to parenthood is a critical period in adult psychological development. Support should be provided to parents who unable to cope, by primary care teams who may refer to telephone help lines, drop-in centres, community support groups and voluntary groups, as well as specialist health and social services. Hence, multidisciplinary training is required to enable primary care professionals to recognize and intervene with parental low self-esteem, anxiety, depression, alcohol and drug misuse. All these factors strongly influence the quality of parental care and infant attachment. This, in turn, increases the risk of child maltreatment and development in the child of poor internal models of relationships and feelings of low self-worth.

Secondary prevention

Secondary prevention involves targeting resources to families identified as being 'high priority' for additional services. The aim of the 'risk approach' of proactive surveillance is to identify children at risk and offer health services and referral to social services before maltreatment occurs. Such an approach has the potential to prevent victimization from ever beginning. Again, primary care professionals and teachers provide the first point of contact with the child and can be alert to signs of potential child maltreatment. For example, doctors and/or community nurses make home visits to monitor child health. At the same time they have the opportunity to screen for socio-demographic and psychological risk factors for child abuse and neglect, classifying families as 'high priority' or 'low priority' for social service referral and/or health service input (e.g. substance misuse programmes or mental health care).

Table 20.2 presents a list of risk factors that has been evaluated on a birth population of 14, 252 new-borns in Surrey, England (Browne and Saqi 1988a). Families with newborns were followed-up over a five-year period and 106 families were suspected of maltreating their child and child protection conferences were called. The prevalence of risk factors in this group of 106 abusing families was compared to the remainder of the birth cohort (14, 146). A greater percentage of abusing families were experiencing each risk factor compared to the non-abusing families. Therefore, each characteristic makes a significant contribution to the chances of child abuse and neglect occurring in the family. The relative contribution was determined by calculating the conditional probability (i.e. the percentage of families with a particular characteristic that later abuse and/or neglect the newborn). A history of family violence (usually spouse abuse) was the most predictive risk factor, which reflects the

Table 20.2 Relative importance of screening characteristics for child abuse as determined by discriminate function analysis (from Browne and Herbert, 1997)

Checklist characteristics	Abusing families	Non-abusing families	Conditional probability*
n = parents with a child under five (baseline)	(n = 106)	(n = 14,146)	0.7%
History of family violence	30.2%	1.6%	12.4%
Parent indifferent, intolerant or over-anxious towards child	31.1	3.1	7.0
Single or separated parent	48.1	6.9	5.0
Socio-economic problems such as unemployment	70.8	12.9	3.9
History of mental illness, drug or alcohol addiction	34.9	4.8	5.2
Parent abused or neglected as a child	19.8	1.8	7.6
Infant premature, low birth weight	21.7	6.9	2.3
Infant separated from mother for more than 24 hours post delivery	12.3	3.2	2.8
Mother less than 21 years old at time of birth	29.2	7.7	2.8
Step-parent or cohabitee present	27.4	6.2	3.2
Less than 18 months between birth of children	16.0	7.5	1.6
Infant mentally or physically disabled	2.8	1.1	1.9

* Conditional probability (in percentages) refers to the percentage of families with a particular characteristic that go on to abuse and/or neglect their newborn in the first five years of life.

established link between spouse abuse and child abuse (Browne and Hamilton 1999). However, Browne (1995a) outlines the dangers of using a one-off screening instrument based on a checklist of risk factors around the time of birth, which can create high numbers of false positives (i.e. identified high risk, but non-maltreating). Browne (1995b) went on to recommend additional behavioural observations that might assist in separating the false positives from the potential cases (i.e. identified high risk and later maltreating – 'hits').

Therefore, Browne and Herbert (1997) describe additional assessments that go beyond a simple risk factor checklist based upon an evaluation of the parent–child relationship. These included:

◆ Caretaker's knowledge and attitudes to parenting the child

◆ Parental perceptions of the child's behaviour and the child's pereption of the parent

◆ Parental emotions and responses to stress

- Style of parent–child interaction and behaviour
- Quality of child to parent attachment
- Quality of parenting

This has led to the development of the CARE programme (Child Assessment and Rating Evaluation) that has been put into practice with community nurses (health visitors) in the Essex area (Browne *et al.* 2000). Initial evaluation on 1,583 families in the Southend Health Care District showed that, using a simple risk factor checklist, 4% of families were identified as a 'high priority', 30% as low priority and 66% as having no risk factors at all. On follow-up it was found that 97% of all parents showed positive parenting skills and only 3% demonstrated insensitive, unrealistic and negative parenting. Those parents with poor skills were significantly more likely to have come from the high priority group. Where both a high number of risk factors and negative parenting existed, these families were regarded as requiring immediate interventions.

The value of home visitation to families with newborns has been highlighted through the work of David Olds (Olds *et al.* 1993, 1997). The research was conducted over a 15-year period and on follow-up a number of significant differences were found between those families visited and those families with newborns who were not. In summary, the visited families showed the following differences:

- Lower rates of child abuse and neglect
- Fewer births after the first child for unmarried women
- Less family aid received
- Fewer problems with alcohol and drugs
- Fewer arrests by police.

These differences were found for both parents and children up to thirteen years after the visitation had ceased. In the first two years, a net dividend of 180 US dollars per family was realized when the cost of the nurse visiting service was compared to savings on Social Welfare provision. Given this evidence-based research, it is surprising to observe a reduction in the community nursing services in the UK. In fact, it could be argued that it would be more cost effective to double the number of community nurses available to families. Nevertheless, it should be recognized that the training of GPs, community psychiatric nurses, health visitors and midwives requires a greater focus on child protection. Without this refocusing, there will be a reliance on tertiary prevention at greater financial and human cost.

Tertiary prevention/intervention strategies

Tertiary prevention is the offering of services to children and families where abuse and/or neglect have already occurred. Reactive surveillance and identification of abused and neglected children leads to intervention both to stop the current maltreatment and to prevent recurrent victimization (Hamilton and Browne 1998). This is an essential service, even in the presence of proactive primary and secondary preventative measures.

It is generally acknowledged that maltreatment of children frequently consists of more than one incident. In a review of 45 studies, DePanfilis and Zuravin (1998) report repeat victimization rates of up to 50% in families followed-up over a five year period and up to 85% for families followed for up to 10 years. In England, Hamilton and Browne (1999) studied 400 children referred to ten child protection units, within the 27 month follow-up period, 1 in 4 children (n = 54) were subject to at least one re-referral. Once maltreated, it was found that children were more likely to be maltreated again. The majority of re-referrals (61%) occurred within 330 days of the index referral, with the greatest risk being the first 30 days. Police and Social Services interventions were not associated with re-referral status. Therefore, the findings of the Hamilton and Browne (1999) study would suggest that the actions taken at a tertiary prevention level (once abuse and/or neglect has occurred) are not effective in preventing the recurrent maltreatment of at least a quarter of those children referred. Such findings demonstrate the need to develop more effective strategies to prevent and detect the victimization and repeat victimization of children.

From a primary health care perspective, children and caregivers/parents attending health service facilities can be classified into a priority system of red, yellow and green for the purposes of referral and intervention. This simplified approach has been successful in the management of childhood illnesses in developing countries (WHO 1999b). Table 20.3 highlights red, yellow and green symptoms of child ill-health and injury that require the doctor/nurse to consider the possibility of non-accidental injury, neglect, sexual and physical abuse to the child, when the red and yellow symptoms are present. A child presenting with red and yellow symptoms accompanied by a non-matching and incongruent explanation from the parent (e.g. a child less than three months who has allegedly rolled over and fallen from the table to the floor) raises the likelihood that non-accidental injury, abuse and/or neglect has occurred. Where there is unreasonable delay in seeking help after a serious injury or illness, which could not be explained by social isolation and distance from the health facility, this would also raise the likelihood of abuse and neglect. Therefore, these questions are incorporated into 'best practice' history taking (see Appendix 1). Green symptoms are reassuring to the health professional in that their presence reduces the possibility of child ill health and maltreatment.

When child abuse and neglect and/or non-accidental injury are suspected and red symptoms are present, this should lead to an emergency referral to specialists in order to determine whether child maltreatment has occurred and if immediate interventions are necessary. When yellow symptoms are present and child abuse and neglect and/or non-accidental injury is suspected, such cases require continued assessments and home-based observation of the family. When only green symptoms are present, standard health service provision should be followed. In the event that red or yellow symptoms coexist with green symptoms, then this indicates that there are some protective factors present and the prognosis for change and rehabilitation is hopeful rather than poor (in the absence of green symptoms). Table 20.4 outlines potential strategies for responding to red, yellow and green symptoms.

Table 20.3 Red and yellow symptoms of child ill-health and injury which require the doctor/nurse to consider the possibility of child abuse and neglect, especially when accompanied by incongruent explanations and/or unreasonable delay in seeking help. Green symptoms are protective factors.

Red symptoms of child

Unconscious, head trauma, floppy, lethargic
Skeletal fractures (old and new)
Chest and abdominal injury
Genital and anal injury or infection
Serious burns and scalds
Severe malnutrition
Child frozen and hyper-vigilant
Child at risk of being abandoned by parent(s)*

Yellow symptoms of child and related parent problems

Multiple cuts and bruises
Minor burns and injuries with inappropriate care and/or poor safety measures
Frequent enuresis and/or encopresis
Disturbed sleep and eating problems
Poor physical hygiene
Little or no immunization
Low height/weight for age
Developmental delay, reduced muscle tone
Child aggressive and anti-social
Parent* depressed/anxious, mentally ill, addicted
Parent* discloses family violence
Parent* constantly criticizes child

Green symptoms of child and parent that protect children

Height and weight within 'normal range'
Progressive physical and psychological development with age
Child shows concern when separated from parent
Child smiles and seeks interaction on reunion
Parental* care and discipline; age appropriate for child and flexible
Parent* interacts and plays sensitively and consistently with the child
Parent* praises child more than criticizes/rebukes

---

* Parent or substitute parent/caregiver

Conclusion

The above recommendations may be rather too simplistic for the sophisticated child protection systems that exist in North America, Western Europe and Australasia. However, such an approach may be useful for training health professionals and, in particular, GPs in thinking more deeply about child protection issues. Due to a number of factors, only 16% of GPs regard attendance at child protection conferences as essential (Simpson *et al.* 1994). In a review of 200 consecutive child protection conferences, there was no primary care team input (attendance or written report) by either the GP or the health visitors in 32% of cases and only 10.5% of child protection conferences were attended by GPs.

Table 20.4 Intervention strategies for responding to red, yellow and green symptoms where there is also a suspicion that child maltreatment has occurred

Red
Very severe to life threatening
Child:
Refer child urgently to hospital care and shelter
Specialist identifies maltreatment
No contact with abuser
Emergency legal care of child
Parents:
Consider subsititute parental care (e.g. fostering or adoption)
Assess rehabilitatiion of non-abusive parent and child
Separation of violent offender
Criminal proceedings?
Yellow
Moderate to less severe
Child:
Family referral to social services and specialist health services
Child remains in family home with one or both parents (assess risk)
Child subject of multidisciplinary case conference
Parent:
Assess rehabilitation of good enough parenting
Closely supervise parents with daily home visits
Specialist psychological support and treatment, assess change
Green
No evidence of abuse or neglect
Child:
Child safe with both parents
Offer health checks and refer if necessary
Parents:
Praise and reinforce positive parenting skills
Review on next contact at health facility, follow up annually

Ideas for engaging GPs in child protection training have been offered by Hendry (1997), but she acknowledges that despite increased efforts and postgraduate educational allowance GP attendance at child protection events is disappointing. Bannon *et al.* (1999) suggest a fresh approach, using primary health care teams as a focus for the development of training in this area. GPs themselves have identified a desire for training in how to promote child welfare in instances of child maltreatment, whilst protecting themselves from criticism or litigation. There is no legal mandate to report British cases of child abuse and neglect to the police and social services, but there is a clear expectation that doctors 'must refer these concerns to the statutory agencies' (Department of Health, British Medical Association, Conference of Medical Royal Colleges 1994).

Nevertheless, any involvement of health professionals in child protection work must be seen in the broader context of multidisciplinary networking and referral processes. For the future development of child protection systems worldwide and for a more effective, less costly system in those countries with a system in place (including the UK), the following WHO Guidelines for Child Protection Best Practice (1999a) require implementation and evaluation.

- Clear policies, protocol and programmes
- Data collection, monitoring and evaluation
- Coordinated and comprehensive services for victims and offenders
- Training and provision of a child friendly approach
- Prevention strategies with families, parents and caretakers e.g. home visits
- Community-based intervention and support
- Interdisciplinary and multi-sector approaches involving policy makers
- International collaboration and partnership.

The prevention of child abuse and neglect in the future is based on the implementation of the UN Convention on the Rights of the Child (1989). This requires all member states to offer effective child protection services. placing the rights of the child and their best interests above those of adults, including the child's own parents. This notion is reflected in the Children Act, 1989, which considers the child's welfare as paramount.

References

Bannon MJ, Carter YH, Barwell F and Hicks C (1999) Perceptions held by General Practitioners in England regarding their training needs in child abuse and neglect. *Child Abuse Review* 8: 276–83.

Bowlby J (1969) *Attachment and Loss, Vol. 1: Attachment*. London: Hogarth.

Browne and KD (1995a) Preventing child maltreatment through community nursing. *Journal of Advanced Nursing* 21: 57–63.

Browne KD (1995b) The prediction of child maltreatment, in P Reder, C Lucey (eds) *Assessment of Parenting: Psychiatric and Psychological Contributions*. London: Routledge.

Browne KD and Hamilton CE (1999) Police recognition of links between spouse abuse and child abuse. *Child Maltreatment* 4(5): 136–47.

Browne KD and Lynch M (1995) The nature and extent of child homicide and fatal abuse (Editorial in special issue on fatal child abuse). *Child Abuse Review* 4: 309–16.

Browne KD and Saqi S (1988a) Approaches to screening families high-risk for child abuse, in KD Browne, C Davies, P Stratton (eds) *Early Prediction and Prevention of Child Abuse*. Chichester: Wiley.

Browne KD and Saqi S (1988b) Mother-infant interactions and attachment in physically abusing families. *Journal of Reproduction and Infant Psychology* 6: 163–82.

Browne KD, Hamilton CE, Heggarty J and Blissett J (2000) Identifying need and protecting children through community nursing home visits. *Representing Children* 13(2): 111–23.

Browne KD and Herbert M (1997) *Preventing Family Violence*. Chichester: J. Wiley.

Cassidy J and Shaver PR (1999) *Handbook of Attachment: Theory, Research and Clinical Applications*. New York: Guilford Press.

Componelle THA (1996) Recognition of child abuse and neglect. *Tjidschhr Kindergeneeskd* **64**: 168–79.

Depanfilis D and Zuravin SJ (1998) Rates, patterns and frequency of child maltreatment recurrences among families known to CPS. *Child Maltreatment* **3**(1): 27–42.

Department of Health (1995) *Child Protection: Messages From Research*. London: HMSO.

Department of Health (1999) *Working Together to Safeguard Children: New Government Proposals for Interagency Co-operation (Social Care Group Consultation paper)*. London: Department of Health Children's Services Branch.

Department of Health (2000) *Children and Young People on Child Protection Registers Year Ending 31ˢᵗ March 2000, England (Personal Social Services and Local Authority Statistics)*. London: Government Statistical Service.

Department of Health, British Medical Association, Conference of Medical Royal Collages (1994) *Child Protection: Medical Responsibilities (Addendum to Working Together Under the Children Act 1989)*. London: Department of Health.

Department of Health, Department of Education and Employment and the Home Office (2000) *Framework for the Assessment of Children in Need and their Families*. London: The Stationery Office.

Hallet C and Birchall E (1992) *Co-ordination and Child Protection*. London: HMSO.

Hamilton CE and Browne KD (1998) The repeat victimisation of children: should the concept be revised? *Aggression and Violent Behavior* **3**(1): 47–60.

Hamilton CE and Browne KD (1999) Recurrent maltreatment during childhood: a survey of referrals to Police Child Protection Units in England. *Child Maltreatment* **4**(4): 275–86.

Hendry E (1997) Engaging General Practitioners in child protection training. *Child Abuse Review* **6**(1): 60–4.

Maccoby EE (1980) *Social Development: Psychology Growth and the Parent-Child Relationship*. New York: Harcourt Brace Jovanovich.

Morton N and Browne KD (1998) Theory and observation of attachment and its relation to child maltreatment: a review. *Child Abuse and Neglect* **22**(11): 1093–104.

National Commission of Enquiry in the Prevention of Child Abuse (1996) *Childhood Matters, Vol 1 and 2*. London: NSPCC.

Olds DL, Henderson CR, Phelps C, Kitzman H and Hanks C (1993) Effect of prenatal and infancy nurse home visitation on Government spending. *Medical Care* **31**(2): 155–74.

Olds D, Eckenrode J, Henderson C, Kitzman H, Powers J, Cole R, Sidora K, Morris P, Pettitt L and Luckey D (1997) Long-term effects of home visitation on maternal life course and child abuse and neglect: fifteen year follow up of a randomized trial. *Journal of the American Medical Association (JAMA)* **278**(8): 637–43.

Simpson CM, Simpson RJ, Power KG, Salter A and Williams G-J (1994) GPs' and health visitors' participation in child protection case conferences. *Child Abuse Review* **3**(3): 211–30.

Simpson JA and Rholes WS (1998) *Attachment Theory and Close Relationships*. New York: Guilford Press.

Sluckin W, Herbert M and Sluckin A (1983) *Maternal Bonding*. Oxford: Blackwell.

Solomon J and George C (1999) *Attachment Disorganization*. New York: Guilford Press.

World Health Organisation (1998a) *First Meeting on Strategies for Child Protection*, Padua, Italy 29–31 October 1998. Copenhagen: WHO Regional Office for Europe.

World Health Organisation (1998b) *Essential Antenatal, Perinatal and Postpartum Care*. Copenhagen: WHO Regional Office for Europe.

World Health Organisation (1999a) *Report of the Consultation on Child Abuse Prevention,* WHO, Geneva, 29–31 March 1999. Geneva: WHO.

World Health Organisation (1999b) *Integrated management of childhood illness* (IMCI information). Geneva: WHO.

Appendix 1

(Adapted from Compenolle, 1996)

Child Protection Questionnaire for Emergency Room (ER)/First Aid Departments

Name (person who fills this in)
Function: Date:

Details of trauma/injury to child

1.   *Who* brings the child to the ER, relationship to the child?
2.   *What kind* of trauma/injury (cut, fracture, firearm wound)?
3.   *Where is the place* of the trauma/injury on the child's body (point out on drawing)?
3a)   Is this the usual place for this sort of trauma/injury?
      Yes   No
4.   How does the trauma/injury look (e.g., colour, form, edges)?
4a)   Does it look like it should?
      Yes   No
5.   When did the accident happen?
      How long ago?
      Time?
5a)   Does this match how it looks?
      Yes   No
6.   What was the cause of the trauma/injury?
7.   What is the story told?
7a)   Does the story explain the place, location and this sort of trauma/injury?
      Doubtful   Yes   No
8.   Who caused the trauma/injury?
8a)   Did he/she come to the ER?
      Yes   No
9.   Which other people saw the accident?
9a)   Did any witnesses come to the ER?
      Yes   No
10.   What actions were taken by the parents, care-takers, others?
10a) Were these actions adequate?
      Yes   No
10b) If not, why not?
11.   Did you find any signs of old traumas?

Child Protection Questionnaire *(continued)*

11a) Did you look for them?

     Yes   No

11b) Did you see them?

     Yes   No

11c) Did you suspect child abuse?

     Yes   No

11d) Did you suspect neglect?

     Yes   No

12. What did you do?

12a) To whom did you refer?

Index